THE

BOOK OF

HEALTHY TEAS

Erika Dillman

THE LITTLE BOOK OF HEALTHY TEAS

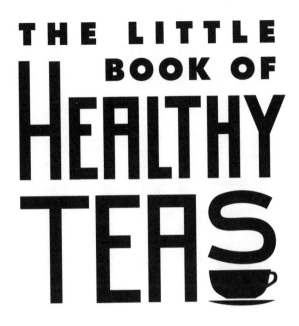

ERIKA DILLMAN

WARNER BOOKS

An AOL Time Warner Company

PUBLISHER'S NOTE: The information herein is not intended to be a substitute for medical advice. You are advised to consult with your health care professional with regard to matters relating to your health, and in particular regarding matters that may require diagnosis or medical attention.

Warner Books, Inc., 1271 Avenue of the Americas, New York, NY 10020

Visit our Web site at www.twbookmark.com.

 An AOL Time Warner Company

Printed in the United States of America
First Printing: March 2002
10 9 8 7 6 5 4 3 2 1

Library of Congress Cataloging-in-Publication Data

Dillman, Erika.
   The little book of healthy teas / Erika Dillman.
      p. cm.
   ISBN 0-446-67728-0
   1. Tea. I. Title.

TX817.T3 D55 2001
641.3'372—dc21   2001046846

Cover design by Rachel McClain
Book design and text composition by L&G McRee
Text illustrations by Jim Chow

For my grandmother
Hanna Anderson

Acknowledgments

I would like to thank my agent, Anne Depue; my editor, Diana Baroni; and assistant editor, Molly Chehak, for their continued support and enthusiasm for my books.

Special thanks to all of the researchers and tea experts who so generously shared their time and expertise with me: Lester A. Mitscher, Ph.D., Kansas University Distinguished Professor, Department of Medicinal Chemistry, University of Kansas; Roderick H. Dashwood, Ph.D., Associate Professor, Environmental and Molecular Toxicology, Linus Pauling Institute, Oregon State University; Craig Foster, Research Manager, Good Earth Teas; Josef Brinckmann, Research and Development Manager, Traditional Medicinals; Brian Keating and the staff of the Teacup tea shop in Seattle, Washington; Bill Waddington of the TeaSource tea shop in St. Paul, Minnesota; Joe Simrany, president of the Tea Council of the USA; and the Tea Council, Ltd. (UK).

Contents

It's Tea Time

*"It is proper for both Winter and Summer, preserving in
    perfect health until extreme old age,
it maketh the body active and lusty...
it removeth lassitude and cleanseth acrid humours..."*

THOMAS GARRAWAY,
seventeenth-century tea trader

Throughout history, tea has relaxed, soothed, and nourished
people around the world. From its earliest uses in ancient
China, where tea was drunk by emperors and used medicinally,
to the tea rooms of England and Europe, where taking tea be-

came a social event as well as a meal, to tea's current status as a healthy, trendy "new" beverage, tea has never failed to delight and intrigue us.

Tea master Sen Rikyu (1522–1591) said, "First you heat the water, then you make the tea. Then you drink it properly. That is all you need to know." Perhaps it is tea's simplicity that we revere. Somehow the combination of hot water and tea leaves creates an aura of magic and mystery, and tea transcends the beverage in the cup and becomes a way of being.

Ninth-century Chinese poet Wangyu-cheng described this phenomenon as a form of self-realization, his precious tea "flooding his soul like a direct appeal, that its delicate bitterness reminded him of the aftertaste of a good counsel." Ancient ideals about tea endure today: to savor a cup is to slow down, step out of the fast-paced world, and take the time to absorb a bit of wisdom.

We've always known that drinking tea makes us feel good, and now scientists are confirming what folk wisdom has professed all along: Tea heals. Researchers in Japan, China, North America, and Europe have discovered that tea, particularly green tea, contains powerful plant chemicals (called phytochemicals) that show great potential in preventing heart disease and cancer, as well as promoting health throughout the body.

Between the stress of modern life and today's promising tea research, there's never been a better time to drink tea. In *The Little Book of Healthy Teas* you'll learn about the history of tea and tea rituals from around the world, the different types of teas, the many health benefits of drinking tea, how to use herbal teas to find relief from the symptoms of common ailments, and how to buy, store, and brew the perfect "cuppa."

There are countless types and varieties of wonderful teas available. This book is for anyone who enjoys tea (or who would like to try tea) and for people interested in finding out more about the health benefits of drinking tea.

Before you begin reading, may I suggest making yourself a nice cup of tea?

ERIKA DILLMAN

1 | *Camellia Sinensis:* The Source of All Tea

"I am in no way interested in immortality, but only in the taste of tea."

LU T'UNG,
eighth-century poet and tea master

After water, tea is the most consumed beverage in the world. It's drunk hot, cold, plain, with sugar, with milk, and in the Himalayas with yak butter. It's stimulating in the morning, reviving in the afternoon, and relaxing at bedtime.

With thousands of teas from which to choose, there's a tea for every taste and every occasion. Black or green, strong or weak, sweet or bitter, dark or light, they all come from one plant, *Camellia sinensis*.

THE TEA BUSH

Camellia sinensis, a shrublike evergreen plant, is grown in tropical climates that provide a combination of hot and cool temperatures and heavy rainfall. Tea plants can be grown at sea level, but the best teas are cultivated at altitudes between 3000 and 7000 feet. Wild tea bushes grow to 50 feet or more; commercially grown tea plants are pruned to about four or five feet high so that pickers can reach the top leaves.

Like fine wine, the quality, flavor, and aroma of tea is influenced by its surroundings. Soil, climate, temperature, rainfall, and altitude all contribute to the unique characteristics of each plant and leaf.

Although tea is now grown in about fifty countries, the finest teas are grown on tea estates or plantations, called gardens, in China, Taiwan (Formosa), Japan, India, and Sri Lanka (Ceylon). Cameroon, Kenya, and Nepal also produce high-quality teas.

TOP TEN TEA-PRODUCING COUNTRIES WORLDWIDE

1. India
2. China
3. Sri Lanka (Ceylon)
4. Kenya
5. Turkey
6. Indonesia
7. Japan
8. Iran
9. Argentina
10. Bangladesh

(Source: ITC Annual Bulletin of Statistics, 2000—
Table B, based on 1999 figures)

TYPES OF TEA

There are five categories of tea: black, oolong, green, white, and pu'erh, which all come from the *Camellia sinensis* plant. Each tea category is determined by the type of processing tea leaves undergo once harvested. Tea is also classified, and often named, by the country and region in which it grows.

More than 2000 varietals, or subspecies, of the tea plant exist in the various growing regions, resulting in thousands of teas, each with unique characteristics. Teas are sold as "single estate" when the tea comes from only one source, or as a blend when two or more types of tea leaves from different estates, regions, or even countries are combined to make a new tea. Flavored teas are black or green teas combined with natural or artificial flavors like mint, spices, honey, mangoes, peaches, and kiwi. Earl Grey is an example of a flavored tea; it's made from black tea and bergamot oil.

> "There are few hours in life more agreeable than the hour dedicated to the ceremony known as afternoon tea."
>
> HENRY JAMES

THE HARVEST

Tea is still harvested the same way it was thousands of years ago—by hand. Pickers, usually women wearing large baskets on their backs, work their way along rows of tea plants, picking leaves according to a "plucking" system. Most tea is gathered by a "coarse plucking," in which the bud and top three or four leaves of a branch are picked. Higher-quality tea requires a "fine plucking," in which just the bud and top two leaves, still young

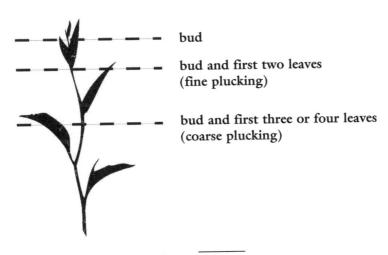

bud

bud and first two leaves
(fine plucking)

bud and first three or four leaves
(coarse plucking)

and fresh, are removed. Premium teas are made from only the downy bud and first leaf of a branch. The gathering method for these teas is called an "imperial plucking."

In ancient China white tea, the purest tea, in which only the downy bud is plucked, was served only to emperors. Today it remains a rare and very expensive type of tea known almost exclusively to connoisseurs.

After the harvest, leaves are processed to produce the five main categories of tea.

MAKING BLACK TEA

Fresh from picking, leaves undergo five stages of very careful processing to become black tea. During withering, the first stage, leaves are spread on a rack or mesh screen and allowed to dry for up to twenty-four hours. Some companies use a machine to speed this process by several hours. This step reduces the moisture content of the leaves by one half, softening the leaves so that they can be rolled. Next, leaves are rolled by hand or machines to release essential oils. Only hand rolling allows the leaf tips to remain intact. Rolled leaves are then placed on mats and sorted into different grades according to size and types (whole or broken). (For a complete breakdown of the different classes of black tea, see chapter 6, page 134.)

In the fourth stage, fermentation (the term "fermentation" actually refers to oxidation, since the process does not yield alcohol), the rolled leaves are placed on tiled floors and tables in a humid, temperature-controlled room for one to three hours. The temperature is kept between 72° and 82° F so that the tea can heat up, then cool. If the air is too warm, the tea will have a burnt flavor, and if it's too cold, it halts the oxidation process. It takes a skilled tea maker to know how to time and judge when to stop this stage.

Next, the leaves are dried or fired in large, hot pans or in drying machines to stop fermentation (i.e., oxidation). Again, timing and skill determine the outcome of the leaves. Finally, the tea is packed and shipped to tea companies.

Generally, black tea produces a dark red or brown liquid and has a smooth, strong taste. Depending on how tea is brewed and on the amount of tea used per cup, black teas generally contain about half the caffeine of coffee. A six-ounce cup of tea contains about 40 to 50 mg of caffeine.

*"Ecstasy is a glass full of tea and
a piece of sugar in the mouth."*

ALEXANDER PUSHKIN

DRINKING BLACK TEAS

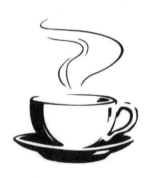

Tea characteristics can vary from harvest
to harvest, region to region, and even
between tea estates within a region. The
following chart, which lists general descriptions of common appearance, taste,
and aroma characteristics, will help you become more familiar
with some of the most common black teas. Similar charts will
follow the descriptions of oolong, green, white, and pu'erh
teas.

As you review these charts, please keep in mind that taste is
a subjective experience and that the descriptions here are very

brief. There's a whole world of tea out there. Sampling many teas is the best way to find your favorites.

Name	Origin	Characteristics
Assam	Assam, India	This tea-growing region produces more tea than any other similar-size geographical area in the world. A strong, hearty, robust, full-bodied tea with a malty flavor. Perfect for breakfast and takes milk well.
Ceylon	Ceylon (Sri Lanka)	When Ceylon gained independence from England and renamed itself Sri Lanka, its government retained the Ceylon name to describe and label its teas. There are two primary types of Ceylons: a crisp light- to medium-bodied tea and a medium- to heavy-bodied tea, characterized by a pronounced sweet, ripe-fruit flavor. Served for breakfast or afternoon tea. Takes milk well.

Name	Origin	Characteristics
Darjeeling	Darjeeling, India	Called the "champagne" of teas, Darjeelings are the highest grown teas in the world (4000–8000 feet). Light body and golden or amber in color, Darjeelings can have a sweet muscat (grape) flavor or a more crisp astringent flavor. Served in the afternoon without milk. Requires the most precision in steeping.
Keemun	China	The original English breakfast tea, also referred to as the "burgundy" of teas, keemuns are deep, rich, black teas with an earthy sweetness and a hint of smokiness. Can be served with milk, but not the higher grades.
Kenyan	Kenya	Hearty, strong black breakfast tea. Great with milk and sugar. Generally machine processed.

Camellia Sinensis: The Source of All Tea

———

Name	**Origin**	**Characteristics**
Lapsang souchong	China	One of the world's most famous teas, this black tea is smoked over pine fires. A strong tea with a smoky, tarry aroma and flavor. Can be served with or without milk. Winston Churchill took his with Scotch.
Nilgiri	India	One of the best values in black tea. Nilgiris are smooth, medium-bodied teas with just a hint of sweetness. Served with or without milk. Simple to steep as inaccurate timing won't ruin the brew.
Russian caravan	China	This blended tea is a milder version of a Lapsang souchong, with a hint of smokiness.
Yunnan	China	Strong, smooth tea with a velvety, al-most silky texture and lingering taste.

———

OOLONG TEA

Oolong tea falls in between black and green tea in terms of processing, taste, and other characteristics, and as a result, shares qualities of black and green teas. During processing, the withering and fermentation (i.e., oxidation) stages are combined, and last only four or five hours rather than the twenty-four-hour fermentation process used to make black tea. Then the leaves are fired to halt fermentation, sorted, and packed. This process results in semifermented tea that contains less caffeine than black tea. Below are a few types of oolong teas from China and Taiwan.

Name	Origin	Characteristics
Formosa oolong	Formosa (Taiwan)	Smooth, medium-bodied with a hint of ripe fruit taste, golden amber liquid.
Wuyi	China	Lighter in color than Formosa oolong, with a hint of green peeking through the amber. Floral flavor.

Name	Origin	Characteristics
Ti Kuan Yin	China	Not as dark as Formosa oolong with a floral flavor.

GREEN TEA

Green tea is made from unfermented tea leaves. Immediately after picking, leaves are panfired in a large metal wok or steamed to break down the enzymes in the leaf that cause fermentation. Panfiring also softens the leaves for rolling. Next, leaves are rolled, then dried, sorted, and packed. This process generally takes twenty-four hours or less.

Because green tea is the least processed tea, except for white tea, more of the tea leaf's beneficial properties remain intact. Green tea has half the caffeine of black tea and varies widely in appearance and taste. Some green teas are light, mild tasting, and pale green or yellow in color. Others can have a bitter or grassy taste. Matcha, the strong tea used in Japanese tea ceremonies, is characterized by its frothy jade liquid. Most of the world's green teas come from Japan, which produces only green teas, and China, which produces black, oolong, and green teas. Below are several well-known green teas.

Name	Origin	Characteristics
ChunMee	China	Also called "precious eyebrows." Light green (with a hint of golden hue) liquid with a sweet, musty taste.
Dragonwell	China	Also called "dragon's well." Yellowish green liquid with a sweet grassy taste.
Gen mai cha	Japan	Some call this "popcorn tea." Blended with roasted and puffed brown rice, it has a roasty, toasty flavor like popcorn.
Gunpowder	China	Named for the appearance of the individually rolled leaves, which resemble pellets or gunpowder. A strong-bodied green tea with hints of sweet and earthy flavors. Medium color green liquid.

Camellia Sinensis: The Source of All Tea

———

Name	Origin	Characteristics
Gyokuro	Japan	Also called "precious dew," this is the finest tea made in Japan. The leaves are a very deep green and, once brewed, produce a luminescent liquid, light green in color. A sweet taste with hints of the sea.
Hojicha	Japan	Made from toasted green tea leaves, it produces an amber or light brown liquid. Hojicha has the most body for a green tea, with a taste reminiscent of almost burnt toast.
Hyson	China	Small, slightly curled green/gray leaves. An earthy, medium-bodied tea.
Matcha	Japan	Thick, frothy, bitter, bright green. Used in traditional Japanese tea ceremonies.

Name	Origin	Characteristics
Pi Lo Chun	China	Also called "green snail spring" or "astounding fragrance." Small leaves curled like snail shells. Tea has a pronounced sweet flavor and aroma.
Sencha	Japan	Fresh taste, pale green, relaxing afternoon tea, with a hint-of-the-sea taste.

WHITE TEA

The purest of all teas, white tea is made from the fresh downy buds of the *Camellia sinensis* bush. White tea is the least processed and rarest of teas, drunk primarily by tea connoisseurs. You won't find white teas at the supermarket, only at fine specialty tea shops. A premium white tea like Yin Zhen (silver needles) can cost $120 or more a pound.

Name	Origin	Characteristics
Yin Zhen	China	Also called "silver needles." The most exotic and expensive tea, harvested by the imperial plucking method.
Pai Mu Tan	China	Smooth, mellow, flowery taste made from large leaves.

PU'ERH TEA

Originally produced in China's Yunnan Province and named after the ancient trading town of Pu-er, Pu'erh tea is a favorite in China. In Yunnan, Pu'erh is considered a medicinal tea, drunk with or after a meal to aid digestion. It is also believed to reduce cholesterol. Pu'erh is the only tea that is aged before processing and whose taste improves with age. Premium pu'erh teas are aged from twenty to sixty years. This mystery tea is processed under vigilant security and secrecy. Nobody outside of its manufacturers in China knows exactly what makes this tea so remarkable. In fact, during the Ming Dynasty (1368–1644) trespassers caught on the plantation were executed.

Name	Origin	Characteristics
Pu'erh	China	Dark black tea with smooth, rich, earthy (peaty) flavor.

HERBAL TEAS (TISANES)

Technically speaking, herbal teas, called "tisanes" in Europe (tisane is the French word for infusion), are not considered true teas since they are made from dried herbs and do not contain tea leaves. However, for simplicity, all of the warm beverages mentioned in this book will be referred to as "teas."

Like tea, herbal teas have been consumed for centuries as healing tonics and traditional medicines. Their use as refreshing beverages is a relatively recent development, and in Germany, where pharmaceutical-quality herbal teas are sold as over-the-counter drugs, 60 percent of packaged teas are medicinal teas. Peppermint, chamomile, and ginger are just a few types of herbal teas. (See chapter 5 for more information on herbal teas.)

ROBUST ROOIBOS: THE REDBUSH TEA

Rooibos tea (pronounced "roy-boss"), grown only in South Africa, shares the best qualities of black and herbal teas. This herbal tea resembles strong black teas in appearance and flavor, but it is naturally caffeine-free, low in tannins (a type of polyphenol in black tea responsible for its sometimes bitter taste), and, like tea, a source of vitamins, minerals, and disease-fighting antioxidants. Rooibos is sometimes referred to as "red-bush tea" (not to be confused with red-colored tea consumed in China). Honeybush tea is another herbal tea grown in South Africa.

"Its liquor is like the sweetest dew from Heaven."
Lu Yu (715–803), poet and tea master

A HEALTHY BREW

With no calories*, fat, or sodium, tea is the ideal healthy drink. Black tea contains half the caffeine of coffee and is a rich source of potassium and manganese. Green tea contains even less caffeine than black tea. Tea also contains several B vitamins, carotene, vitamin C, folic acid, iron, fluoride, and calcium.

In its simplest application, tea can relax or revive, providing relief from stress, headaches, and indigestion. Research has shown that tea contains powerful phytochemicals called polyphenols, which act as antioxidants in the body. Antioxidants, which are also found in fruits and vegetables, help maintain and protect healthy cells and tissues.

Scientists are studying tea's antioxidants to determine their potential for promoting health and protecting against serious diseases.

*Tea does contain organic matter and may have up to three to four calories per one-cup serving.

2 | A World of Tea

"There is a great deal of poetry and fine sentiment in a chest of tea."

RALPH WALDO EMERSON

According to legend, tea was discovered in China almost 5000 years ago by Emperor Shen Nung when a tea leaf fell into a pot of water he was boiling. The rest, as they say, is history.

Originally valued for its medicinal properties, tea became the drink of emperors, aristocrats, and eventually, of the common man. Tea has held a place in our collective consciousness and daily lives for so long that everyone has a favorite tea and every culture has its own unique tea rituals and ceremonies.

ALL THE TEA IN CHINA

For millennia, tea has been entwined with China's history, social customs, and economy. From its earliest uses in religious ceremonies and as a digestive aid and stimulant, tea, made by boiling wild camellia leaves in water, evolved into a social drink and a valuable trade commodity.

By the Chin Dynasty (A.D. 557–589), tea was used as medicine and also enjoyed for its taste. It was offered to guests as a sign of friendship and hospitality, a custom started by a Buddhist monk who greeted his teacher with a bowl of tea.

In the following decades, tea became a commercially cultivated crop. Tea leaves were harvested, crushed, and pressed into cakes called tea bricks, which were also used as currency in trade. Tea was made by breaking off small pieces of the brick and boiling them in water. This bitter-tasting tea was often flavored with salt, ginger, or onions.

> "Better to be deprived of food for three days than of tea for one."
>
> CHINESE PROVERB

A World of Tea

Tea's popularity soared during the T'ang Dynasty (620–907). Now widely available, tea was universally revered and, for the first time, taxed. Tea growers held harvest festivals, making "offerings" of their best teas to the emperor. As tea became part of daily life, tea masters began to establish the guidelines of the tea ceremony.

One of those tea masters was poet Lu Yu, considered the patron saint of tea, who wrote an encyclopedia of tea called *Ch'A Ching* (Book of Tea) in 780. The book is filled with elaborate descriptions of growing, harvesting, preparing, and serving tea. Yu even described in minute detail the twenty-four essential utensils used in tea ceremonies.

Taoist poet and tea master Lu T'ung, one of Yu's disciples, earned himself the nickname "tea maniac" for his absolute devotion to tea. T'ung lived in seclusion in the mountains of the Hunan Province, drinking tea and writing poetry. His poem "Thanks to Imperial Censor Mêng for His Gift of Freshly Picked Tea" is one of the most well-known tea poems:

...The first drink sleekly moistened my lips and throat;
The second banished all my loneliness;
The third expelled the dullness from my mind,

Including inspirations born from all the books I've read;
The fourth broke me out in a light perspiration,
Disbursing a lifetime's troubles through my pores.
The fifth drink bathed every atom of my being.
The sixth lifted me higher to kinship with Immortals.
This seventh is the utmost I can drink—...

By the Song Dynasty (960–1279), the spread of teahouses, the creation of clay teapots and bowls, and tea contests, where growers competed to make the best tea, all demonstrated tea's rising status in Chinese culture. Tea used in ceremonies was made by whisking dried, powdered tea leaves and hot water to produce a frothy, bright green liquid. Emperor Hui Tsung (1100–1126), a dedicated tea drinker, wrote his own book about tea, *Ta Kaun Ch'a Lun*, which extolled the health benefits of his cherished elixir. The emperor's tea, of course, had to be of the purest quality, harvested by virgins who wore white gloves and used gold scissors to cut the bud and first young leaf.

It wasn't until the Ming Dynasty (1368–1644) that tea growers developed new processing methods that allowed them to make black and oolong teas in addition to their green teas.

THE ZEN OF TEA

Tea was introduced to Japan in A.D. 600 by Buddhist monks, who drank *matcha*, a strong, nourishing powdered green tea, to help them remain alert during long hours of meditation. A Buddhist monk named Saichô brought the first tea plants to Japan from China around the beginning of the ninth century.

Where China had revered tea for its many uses, Japan exalted it to a spiritual practice and art form that personified Zen precepts of harmony, purity, respect, and tranquillity. The tea ceremony, called *chanoyu*, was a strictly disciplined event where host and guest communed over tea. Tea master Sen Rikyu, who outlined the guidelines for "the way of tea," as he referred to the ceremony, described the tea ceremony as a spiritual exercise:

"In Zen, truth is pursued through discipline of meditation in order to realize enlightenment, while in Tea we use training in the actual procedures of making tea to achieve the same end."

Ceremonies took place in a small teahouse called *sukiya*, where everything from the design of the house and surrounding garden to the tea bowls and utensils used in preparing the tea had significance. During the four-hour tea, host and guests shared different types of green tea, as well as a light meal and sweet and savory snacks. Matcha tea, the green, frothy whisked tea drunk in China during the Song Dynasty, was served during the ceremony, along with another, lighter green tea served later in the ceremony.

These tea ceremonies still exist today in Japan and can be found in major cities around the world.

A World of Tea

HOW DO YOU TAKE YOUR TEA?

Country	Custom
China	Black, oolong, or green
Japan	Green
Tibet	Green with salt and yak butter
Russia	Green or black with a spoonful of jam or a sugar cube in the mouth
Egypt	Black, strong and sweet, no milk
Afghanistan	Green or black with sugar
Morocco	Green with mint
Britain and Ireland	Black with milk (and sugar)
South Africa	Rooibos, plain or with milk
India	Black or black with sugar, milk, and spices (called Chai)
United States	Black, iced, with sugar and lemon; black with milk and sugar; green

TRADING TEA

Dutch traders introduced tea to Europe in the sixteenth century. The imported green tea was initially considered a medicinal drink and dispensed by apothecaries. During this time it was also common to drink herbal infusions or decoctions to treat common ailments. By the seventeenth century, tea had become a popular beverage with the upper classes, particularly in Germany, France, and eventually, England. The first public sale of tea in England took place in 1657.

INDIA: ASSAM AND DARJEELING

India's tea history is also Britain's. As tea became more popular, even replacing beer as the favorite drink of Britain's lower classes, China was unable to keep up with the increasing demand. By the 1820s, eager to break China's monopoly on tea, Britain sent botanists, among them James Fortune, into China to learn more about the growth, cultivation, harvest, and processing of tea.

Disguised as a Buddhist monk, Fortune was able to get an

insider's view into the secretive world of China's tea plantations. He visited tea-growing regions around the country and discovered how tea leaves were processed to make black tea. Fortune also learned one of the most important aspects of brewing tea from the Buddhist monks who helped him on his journey: to use the freshest, purest water when making tea. Legend tells of a tea master who could tell the difference between tea made from water drawn from the middle of a river, from its banks, or from a well.

With Fortune's research, Britain began clearing forest areas in India's Assam and Darjeeling regions to establish tea plantations. Today Assam and Darjeeling still produce some of the world's finest black teas.

> "The Way of Tea teaches us the spirit of sincerity and gratitude."
>
> SOSHITSU SEN, Grand Master XV,
> Urasenke School of Tea

THE BRISK TEA

Tea was a minor crop in Ceylon, another British colony, until 1869 when a fungus decimated coffee plants, the nation's major cash crop. Recognizing Ceylon's potential as a tea-producing nation, Thomas Lipton, a British businessman who owned a chain of grocery stores, bought several plantations and quickly transformed Ceylon into one of the world's top tea-growing regions.

Lipton was the first tea grower to streamline the process of manufacturing tea and selling it directly to his customers, eliminating tea brokers and other middlemen.

TEA IN BRITAIN

No country in the western world is associated with a national tea habit more than Great Britain.

As tea drinking became more popular in the eighteenth century, teahouses began to spring up all over London. Where coffeehouses had been open only to men, teahouses were open to both men and women. Eventually tea replaced coffee as the nation's favorite warm drink. Twining's, another British tea company, opened one of the first teahouses in London in 1717. This small tea shop on the Strand is still open today.

More than a habit, tea became part of the national identity. Even Winston Churchill praised tea's virtues when he claimed that tea improved morale among British troops during World War II.

Today in Great Britain, a 4:00 P.M. teatime is strictly observed. Tea is served with milk and sometimes sugar, although the debate continues over whether milk should be added to the cup before or after tea is poured.

TOP TEN TEA-DRINKING NATIONS
(based on per capita consumption)

1. Ireland
2. Turkey
3. Libya
4. United Kingdom
5. Qatar
6. Kuwait
7. Iraq
8. Iran
9. Morocco
10. Sri Lanka (Ceylon)

(Source: U.S. Tea Association, based on 1997–1999 figures)

TEA AMERICAN STYLE

Tea actually arrived, via Dutch traders, in the British colonies in North America before it arrived in England. Popular with all social classes, tea was especially celebrated by the upper classes, who threw lavish tea parties, even buying pure springwater for brewing.

Since most of the tea that came to the colonies was from China, people primarily drank green tea, flavored with sugar, saffron, flower blossoms, or peach leaves. By the mid-1700s, tea was the third major import to the colonies.

Eventually, Britain's East India Company edged out Dutch traders and dominated the tea trade. When Britain needed to raise money to fund the French and Indian War, the East India Company raised taxes on tea, provoking a bitter reaction from colonists. Refusing to pay the higher taxes and asserting their increasing desire for independence from Britain, colonists boycotted tea and trade ships packed with tea remained in port.

On December 16, 1773, colonists rebelled against Britain and made history when a group of men disguised as Native Americans boarded trading ships in Boston Harbor and threw crates of tea overboard. Now referred to as the Boston Tea

Party, this historic event was one of several that led to the creation of the Declaration of Independence.

According to the U.S. Tea Council, 80 percent of the tea consumed in America is iced black tea, which was created in 1904 at the St. Louis World's Fair. An Englishman named Richard Blechynden was at the fair promoting black teas from India. Unfortunately for Mr. Blechynden, the sweltering summer temperatures were not conducive to tea drinking. In desperation, he added ice to cups of tea. People loved it, and a national drink was born.

Although coffee still reigns as the hot beverage of choice, tea is becoming more popular as people learn about the many varieties of tea and its impressive health benefits.

3 | Tea and Health

"Tea tempers the spirit and harmonizes the mind, dispels lassitude and relieves fatigue, awakens thought and prevents drowsiness."

LU YU

It doesn't take a scientist to know that tea can soothe a sore throat, settle an upset stomach, ease the pain of a headache, or simply help you unwind after a long day. Chinese and Japanese cultures have used tea for thousands of years as a healing tonic as well as a refreshing beverage.

Now modern science is taking a closer look at tea's health benefits. Researchers have discovered that tea contains powerful disease-fighting phytochemicals called polyphenols. Many studies have shown that tea, particularly green tea, which contains more powerful polyphenols than black or oolong tea, may have the potential to reduce the risk of the top two major causes of death in this country, heart disease and cancer, when included in a healthy diet.

TEA'S HEALTH BENEFITS

Findings from recent and current tea research looks very promising that tea, in addition to being one of the world's favorite beverages, might also be one of its healthiest. In addition to its soothing effects, tea's antioxidant power makes it an ideal dietary supplement for promoting health and preventing disease.

Here are just a few of tea's health benefits that researchers are studying:

- Tea may reduce the risk of heart disease.
- Tea has the potential to reduce the risk of some types of cancer.
- Tea aids digestion.

- Tea reduces fatigue and improves concentration.
- Tea prevents cavities.
- Tea relaxes and revives body and mind.
- Tea may be helpful in combating arthritis and rheumatism.
- Tea may be helpful as a weight-loss aid.

POWERHOUSE POLYPHENOLS

To understand how tea provides protective effects in the body, let's first take a look at some of the substances in tea, namely, *polyphenols*, *flavonoids*, and *catechins*.

- *Polyphenols*, found in most plants, are the primary sources of tea's potency as a health-promoting, disease-fighting beverage. Tea's polyphenols are more powerful than those found in some fruits and vegetables. Green tea polyphenols are believed to be more powerful than polyphenols in black tea. A recent study at Oregon State University indicated that white tea, the rarest and least processed of teas, may contain the most potent polyphenols of all the teas.

Flavonoids, also found in onions, red grapes, blueberries, and apples, are one type of polyphenol found in tea, and *catechins* are a type of flavonoid. Certain catechins are more powerful in green tea than in black tea due to processing methods used to make black tea.

EGCG (epigallocatechin gallate) is one of the four primary polyphenols, or catechins, in green tea, including *EC* (epicatechin), *ECG* (epicatechin gallate), and *EGC* (epigallocatechin).

Some polyphenols, like the flavonoids and catechins found in tea, function as *antioxidants*, substances in the body that prevent *free radicals* (in other words, unstable molecules) from causing cell damage that can lead to disease and cancer.

AMAZING ANTIOXIDANTS

You've probably heard of antioxidants before, like vitamins C and E, beta-carotene, and coenzyme Q10. Antioxidants play an important role in maintaining health by preventing free radicals from causing cell damage that can lead to illness, aging, and disease and lay the foundation for cancer to develop in the body. Oranges, strawberries, spinach, broccoli, and red peppers are just a handful of the fruits and vegetables containing antioxidants.

Nutritionists, doctors, and scientists recommend a diet high in antioxidant-rich fruits and vegetables (and low in animal products, which contain saturated fat) to help reduce the risk of heart disease and some cancers. In fact, the American Cancer Society suggests that two thirds of cancers can be prevented by improving diet and stopping unhealthy lifestyle habits, especially smoking.

Scientists believe that tea might be a perfect dietary supplement for providing powerful antioxidants. For example, researchers have discovered that green tea contains 200 times the antioxidants as vitamin E, making it 25 times more effective than vitamin E at neutralizing free radicals. Green tea's antioxidant properties may also be 100 times more effective than vitamin C. A study at the University of Nebraska confirmed that the high levels of antioxidant polyphenols found in tea can be absorbed by the body.

"If you are cold, tea will warm you;
if you are too heated, it will cool you;
if you are depressed, it will cheer you;
if you are exhausted, it will calm you."

WILLIAM GLADSTONE,
British Prime Minister, 1865

Tea's flavonoids might be more powerful than antioxidants in some fruits and vegetables. A research study conducted by the United States Department of Agriculture (USDA) showed that in test tube studies (i.e., in vitro studies), the flavonoids in one serving of black or green tea were more effective against one type of free radical than one serving of several different vegetables, including brussels sprouts, broccoli, carrots, and garlic. A similar USDA study revealed that in test tube studies, black and green tea were also more potent at fighting one type of free radical than one serving of different fruits, including grapefruit, apples, grapes, and kiwi.

Before you blow off brussels sprouts for good, remember that drinking tea is not a substitute for eating a well-balanced plant-based diet. Fruits and vegetables contain a variety of important nutrients and other substances that work together to promote and maintain health.

TEA RESEARCH

When comparing disease rates of different countries, scientists look at lifestyle habits and diet to determine possible causes of disease. In some cases, they find that certain countries or regions have lower disease rates than others with similar lifestyles. Researchers call this phenomenon "the French paradox." For many years doctors wondered why France had a relatively low rate of heart disease despite the typical high-fat French diet. The key to France's healthy hearts, it turned out, was red wine, ubiquitous on French dinner tables and a rich source of disease-fighting polyphenols.

Scientists discovered a similar trend in Japan's Shizuoka province, the largest tea-growing region in the country. This area has the lowest death rate from cancer in Japan and reports virtually no incidences of stomach cancer. Researchers believe that the high consumption of green tea (the average is ten small cups a day) in Japan provides protective effects against major diseases like cancer and heart disease. Other examples of this phenomenon are Japan's and China's relatively low lung cancer rates despite both countries' high smoking rates.

These phenomena indicate that there might be some lifestyle or dietary habits that provide protection against common diseases, even in populations where smoking and/or high-fat diets are common. Based on promising epidemiological findings like these, researchers in China, Japan, Europe, Canada, England, and the United States have focused their studies on how tea's polyphenols work in the body to promote health and provide protection against common illnesses and diseases. More than 500 studies have been conducted on green tea alone.

It's worth mentioning here that there's no silver bullet when it comes to maintaining health. Researchers are quick to point out that while tea is a healthy beverage containing disease-fighting substances, drinking tea is not a cure-all or a substitute for medical care or for healthy lifestyle habits like eating a diet rich in plant foods, exercising regularly (the U.S. Department of Health recommends exercising for thirty minutes at moderate intensity almost every day), and not smoking.

Most tea research to date has been epidemiological (i.e., comparing lifestyle habits and disease rates within populations), in vitro, or in vivo (i.e., using animal subjects). Long-term, well-controlled studies using human subjects are the next step in testing the theories about tea's potential to protect human health.

"For tea, though ridiculed by those who are
naturally coarse in their nervous sensibilities,
or are become so from wine-drinking,
and are not susceptible of influence from so refined
a stimulant, will always be the favored beverage
of the intellectual...."

THOMAS DE QUINCEY (1785–1859),
Confessions of an Opium-Eater

HELP YOUR HEART

Epidemiological studies and current research suggest that tea may help prevent heart disease and heart attack by addressing the two primary risk factors for heart disease, high cholesterol levels and high blood pressure. Tea lowers total cholesterol, improves the ratio of LDL to HDL cholesterol, and reduces blood pressure. Some researchers suggest that tea, like aspirin, thins the blood.

Cholesterol is a naturally occurring substance produced by the liver and used in metabolism. It is also found in some foods (i.e., animal products). High-density lipoprotein (HDL), often referred to as the "good" cholesterol, carries cholesterol to the liver, where it is broken down and eventually excreted from the body. Low-density lipoprotein (LDL) carries cholesterol through blood vessels. When cholesterol levels are too high, LDL cholesterol, the "bad" cholesterol, leaves fatty deposits in the blood vessels that clog arteries, damage blood vessels, and reduce blood flow, contributing to atherosclerosis (clogged arteries).

High blood pressure is a problem for one out of four people in the United States, and with the growing rate of obesity in this country, more children are at increased risk. High blood pressure damages blood vessels and also increases stroke risk.

Research looks promising that drinking tea (black or green) is good for heart health, and it appears from several studies that the more tea you drink, the more benefits you gain. Studies have shown that green tea drinkers have a lower incidence of heart disease than non–tea drinkers, men who eat and/or drink flavonoids (which are highly concentrated in tea) reduce their risk of heart disease, and women who drink one to two cups of black tea a day reduce by half their risk of atherosclerosis.

Here are some specific ways that tea promotes health, followed by a list of recent tea research:

1. Flavonoids in tea help reduce blood clotting and prevent cholesterol deposits in arteries.

2. Antioxidants in tea help maintain healthy blood vessels.

3. Antioxidants prevent LDL from becoming oxidized by free radicals.

4. EGCG in green tea blocks the absorption of cholesterol by blood vessels.

Studies have found that:

- Green tea lowers cholesterol. In one study, men who drank green tea reduced their cholesterol levels. Men in the study who drank nine cups of tea a day had lower cholesterol levels than men who drank two cups a day.

- Subjects who drank one or more cups of black tea daily reduced their heart attack risk by 44 percent compared to subjects who did not drink tea.

- Men and women who drank black tea showed decreases in total cholesterol levels and LDL levels and increased levels of HDL.

- Men who drank black tea lowered their cholesterol levels. The men who drank five cups of tea a day lowered their cholesterol levels more than those who drank one cup a day. Women tea drinkers also lowered their cholesterol levels. The study also showed that the more tea people drank, the more their systolic blood pressure lowered. Researchers also concluded that tea drinkers were less likely to die from heart attack than non–tea drinkers.

Drinking one to two cups of black tea a day lowered study subjects' risk of severe coronary artery disease by 46 percent. Drinking four or more cups a day lowered risk by 69 percent. Women in the study benefited from tea's protective effects more than men.

Green tea relaxed blood vessel walls. Subjects who drank green tea (which contains more polyphenols than black tea) demonstrated a 91-percent change in relaxation. Black tea drinkers had a 60-percent change in relaxation.

When mice were placed in stressful situations and then given decaffeinated green tea, their blood pressure dropped.

"Tea is a divine herb. Profits are ample if one plants it.
The spirits are purified if one drinks it.
It is something esteemed by the wellborn and well-to-do
which the plebeians and social dregs also cannot
do without.
Truly it is a necessity in the daily life of man,
and an asset for the fiscal prosperity of the
commonwealth."

XU GUANGQI, statesman (1562–1633),
Book of Agricultural Administration

STOP STROKES

Tea's polyphenols might help prevent strokes by addressing the same primary risk factors as heart disease, high cholesterol, and high blood pressure. Both can lead to atherosclerosis, the most common cause of strokes.

Tea and Health

The relationship between tea and stroke has not been studied as widely as some of the more common diseases like cancer and heart disease, but researchers believe that tea does provide protective effects against stroke risks.

Studies of tea and stroke have shown that:

- Stroke was less common in women who drank green tea than their non–tea-drinking counterparts. When these women were revisited four years later, the women who drank more than five cups of green tea a day had less occurrence of stroke than the non–tea drinkers.

- Men who had the highest intake of flavonoids had a 73 percent lower stroke rate than men who had a low intake of flavonoids (70 percent of the flavonoid source was black tea). Men who drank 4.7 cups a day of black tea had better test results than men who drank 2.6 cups a day.

- Poststroke patients (average age sixty-six) who were given green tea extract as part of their treatment showed improvement.

CURTAIL CANCER

When it comes to cancer prevention, green tea polyphenols have demonstrated the most significant results in animal and in vitro studies.

Cancer develops when there's a breakdown in genetic material that allows rapid and uncontrolled cell growth. Cancer cells are then replicated and can spread throughout the body, resulting in disease that overpowers the immune system and destroys healthy cells, tissues, and organs. Tea's polyphenols work as powerful antioxidants to support the immune system and maintain healthy cells and tissues.

Researchers believe that there are three primary ways in which green tea works to prevent cancer. First, antioxidants stop free radicals from damaging healthy cells and tissue. Green tea's polyphenols also prevent damaged cells from metastasizing (i.e., multiplying and spreading throughout the body). Finally, green tea may halt tumor growth. Scientists are also examining tea's efficacy as a supplement to cancer treatments.

Studies have shown that tea, particularly green tea, helps

prevent many types of cancer (including esophageal, digestive system, colon, lung, prostate, breast, and skin) from developing. Epidemiological evidence shows that Japanese people living in the tea-producing area of Shizuoka, where it's common to drink an average of ten cups of green tea a day, have low cancer rates. (*Note:* Japanese teacups are smaller than the six- to seven-ounce cups typically used in the United States.)

✼✼

"Tea, heav'ns delight, and natures truest wealth, that pleasing physic, and pledge of health, the statesman's counselor, the virgin's love, the muse's nectar, the drink of love."

PETER ANTOINE MOTTEUX,
"A Poem Upon Tea," 1712

✼✼

Cancer is the second leading cause of death in the United States. Some of the top cancer threats to men include prostate, lung, colon and rectum, bladder, and lymphoma. Breast, lung, colon and rectum, uterine, and ovarian cancer top the list for women. According to the American Cancer Society, two thirds of all cancers could be prevented by lifestyle and diet changes, as mentioned earlier in this chapter.

Cancer is a complicated disease, with many causes. Adding tea to an already healthy lifestyle may be a great way to support your immune system, although exercising regularly and not smoking are vitally important for overall good health.

Studies have shown that:

☕ EGCG in green tea blocks the mutation of cells, reducing cell damage; blocks tumor growth; and blocks the liver enzymes that convert pro-carcinogens (i.e., harmless substances in the body that can turn into cancer agents) into carcinogens.

☕ EGCG in green tea blocks enzymes that cause cancer cells to grow and it can destroy cancer cells without damaging surrounding healthy cells. Scientists also revealed that this effect is 10 to 100 times more potent in green tea than in black tea.

- Green tea prevents the initiation stage of cancer (i.e., the mutation of DNA); blocks cell damage from nitrates (i.e., substances in meats that turn carcinogenic when meat is cooked or blackened); and metabolizes carcinogens, rendering them inactive. One study suggested that drinking five cups of tea a day and drinking tea before eating meat may provide protective effects from nitrates.

- Animal studies have shown that white tea protects against early stages of colon cancer in animals.

- Tea increases the blood's antioxidant capacity.

- Based on animal studies, tea may reduce the risk of lung cancer.

☕ EGCG in green tea makes cancer drugs twenty times more effective. Scientists added EGCG to test tubes containing breast cancer cells and the cancer drug tamoxifen. The green tea–enhanced mixture killed twice as many cancer cells as tamoxifen alone.

☕ EGCG kills cancer cells and, in particular, inhibits prostate cancer cells.

☕ Precancerous oral lesions showed significant improvement and decreased proliferation after being treated with a mixture of black and green tea substances.

☕ Green tea has been shown to reduce damage to blood vessels in smokers.

☕ Green tea's polyphenols can boost white blood cells, and might be an effective supplement to chemotherapy and radiation treatments that impact bone marrow and lower white blood cell count.

- Men who drank two to three cups of tea a day reduced their risk of prostate cancer.

- Women who had a history of drinking five or more cups of green tea a day had fewer recurrences of breast cancer and a slower spread of the disease.

- Postmenopausal women who drank two or more cups of tea a day lowered their overall cancer risk by 10 percent and their incidence of digestive and urinary tract cancers by 40 to 70 percent.

- Regular green tea drinkers (who did not smoke or drink alcohol) had a 60-percent lower risk of esophageal cancer than non–tea drinkers.

IMMUNI-TEA

Maintaining a strong immune system is critical to health. Of course, eating a healthy diet and exercising regularly are the most important ways to support the immune system. Drinking tea may be a good supplement for boosting the immune system.

Research has shown that tea's polyphenols boost immune functioning and reduce the impact of foreign microorganisms in the body. (Certainly some of this effect is due to the fact that tea is made with boiling water, which kills many harmful microorganisms in the water.)

Studies have shown that:

● Tea can stop the growth and reproduction of some strains of bacteria that cause diarrhea.

● Tea might help fight illnesses like pneumonia and whooping cough. Tea was shown to fight cholera in animals.

● Green tea exhibits antiviral activity. Animal studies have shown that EGCG interferes with the influenza virus, preventing infection, and that it may provide protection against the HIV virus (more research needs to be done on humans).

TOUGHEN YOUR TEETH, BUILD YOUR BONES

Studies in Britain and Japan suggest that tea protects teeth and bones. A natural source of fluoride, tea (both green and black) may be helpful in preventing tooth decay that leads to cavities. Tea's antioxidants also play a role in oral health by preventing the growth of a bacteria that causes plaque to form on teeth.

According to the British Dental Association, 2½ cups of tea a day provides the recommended daily requirement of fluoride.

In a University of Cambridge School of Medicine study, researchers determined that women who drank tea had higher bone density levels than non-tea drinkers. Women who added milk to their tea had the highest bone density levels.

LIVER AND KIDNEY DETOX

A natural diuretic, tea helps cleanse and detoxify the liver and kidneys. Tea's catechins support liver enzyme functioning and protect the liver from toxins. Epidemiological research from Japan suggests that the more green tea people consume, the less liver damage they exhibit. EGCG is believed to prevent pro-carcinogens in the liver from becoming carcinogens and to protect the liver from some types of toxic mold.

In China, green tea is given to kidney patients along with their prescribed medications. Studies have shown that drinking green tea improves kidney function.

" 'Tea and Water give each other life,'
the Professor was saying.
'The tea is still alive. This tea has tea and water vitality,'
he added. ' . . . Afterwards the taste still happens . . .
It rises like velvet . . . It is a performance.' "

JASON GOODWIN,
The Gunpowder Gardens

DIGESTION AND WEIGHT LOSS

Drinking warm tea stimulates the digestive system and provides diuretic and laxative effects. With only four calories and no fat per cup, tea is an ideal beverage for people watching their weight.

Scientists believe that green tea may help the body digest carbohydrates and regulate carbohydrate absorption so that carbohydrates are released slowly into the bloodstream. This mechanism maintains healthy insulin levels, which encourages the body to burn, not store, fat. If this hypothesis is proven, it could also be an important discovery for diabetics.

SKIN CARE

Green tea's antioxidants protect the body from cell damage caused by free radicals. As a drink or applied topically, green tea has shown promise in preventing some types of skin cancer. In a study conducted at Case Western Reserve, researchers showed that green tea, applied topically or internally, protected mice from cancer caused by UV radiation. Although green tea is beneficial to skin as an astringent and possible wrinkle preventer, the efficacy of skin products containing green tea at providing protective effects has not been determined.

Green tea and rooibos tea have both been used to reduce minor skin irritations and allergies.

A recent study from Rutgers University suggests that skin tumors in mice might be reduced by components in green tea.

TEA FOR A LONG, HEALTHY LIFE

In both China and Japan, drinking tea has been a way of life for thousands of years. Today it remains a national beverage, as well as a medicinal brew. Although many lifestyle factors may account for Asia's lower rates of heart disease and some types of cancer, drinking green tea (and drinking a lot of it) is suspected to play some role in preserving and prolonging life.

Researchers in China have tested this theory by extending

the lives of fruit flies with jasmine tea. A similar experiment in Japan used green tea to extend the lives of rats. A Japanese study of female tea masters, who generally consume above average amounts of green tea, concluded that they did have longer life spans compared to other Japanese women.

A LIFETIME OF TEA

There's no doubt that tea is a healthy beverage. It relaxes, revives, and soothes mind and body, aids in digestion, and provides necessary fluoride to teeth, to name just a few of its health benefits. Tea is also an excellent beverage for replacing fluid in the body as well as a calorie-free substitute for sweetened, carbonated drinks.

Despite promising results from many research studies, long-term health benefits of drinking tea have yet to be confirmed in human health and researchers are not suggesting that tea be used as a medicine. Many factors, including the quality and type of tea used, how long tea is steeped, how tea is processed and stored, and lifestyle habits, influence the beneficial properties of tea and how it may affect health. For these reasons scientists do not recommend specific teas or doses to treat specific illnesses.

A much more useful and simple way to view tea is as a healthy drink that supplements a healthy diet and lifestyle.

4 | Your Cup of Tea

"The effect of tea is cooling. As a drink, it suits very well persons of self-restraint and good conduct. When feeling hot, thirsty, depressed, suffering from headache, eye-ache, fatigue of the four limbs, or pains in the joints, one should drink tea only, four or five times."

LU YU, *Ch'A Ching*, 780

Tea's list of health benefits is certainly impressive, but you might be wondering how all of that research applies to your health. What kind of tea should you drink? Do you have to be a tea maniac like Lu T'ung to reap the benefits of tea?

Thankfully, you can hold off for now on devoting your life to tea. You might want to increase your tea consumption a bit, but drinking tea—for its taste and its healing properties—doesn't require a dramatic lifestyle change. In this chapter you'll learn about some of the healthful aspects of tea so that you can choose your favorite cup of tea.

SAVOR THE FLAVOR

Unlike coffee, which many of us drink on the run, tea can't be rushed. Before you start thinking about how you'll take your tea, don't forget that part of the tea-drinking experience is allowing yourself to slow down and relax, if only for a few minutes, so that you can savor the aroma, flavor, and wisdom in a steaming cup. Try to clear your mind and let the tea warm and calm you. You might be surprised by the restorative powers of taking time out for tea. Even a short break can promote mental and physical relaxation and have beneficial effects on your health and mood.

> "I don't drink coffee; I take tea, my dear."
>
> STING, "An Englishman in New York"

SELECTING A TEA

Your first step in becoming a tea drinker is to find out what types of tea you enjoy drinking. Therefore, the most important criterion for you to consider is taste. Don't worry about finding the "healthiest" tea; the tea that you'll drink the most is the best tea for you. With thousands of varieties available, it shouldn't be hard to find several teas that you like. As you can see in the tea descriptions on pages 9–18, you may find that you prefer some types of tea in the morning and other types of tea in the afternoon.

The best way to learn more about tea is to visit a specialty tea shop with a knowledgeable staff that can help you find which teas you like best. Sample a variety of teas so that you can become more familiar with the different taste characteristics of the five main tea types (black, oolong, green, pu'erh, and white) as well as herbal teas and rooibos tea.

At a reputable tea shop, you'll get a chance to drink tea that has been brewed correctly. Water quality, tea quality, and brewing time all influence taste. For example, if the water used to make green tea is too hot, it can stew the leaves, resulting in a bitter tea. Steeping tea too long or using poor quality tea or water can also alter the taste of tea. It's very common for people to think they don't like a certain type of tea when, in fact, poor preparation has completely changed its taste.

You can take your tea journey one step farther by experiencing "the way of tea" practiced in other countries. There are teahouses and grand hotels across the country that host British-style afternoon teas. For an authentic Japanese *chanoyu* ceremony, contact the Urasenke Foundation to find out if there's a chapter in your city that hosts tea ceremonies. The Urasenke Foundation is based in Kyoto, Japan, and has branches in cities around the world, including Washington, D.C., San Francisco, New York, Seattle, London, Paris, and Zurich.

BLACK, GREEN, WHITE, OR REDBUSH?

All teas made from the *Camellia sinensis* plant contain disease-fighting polyphenols. If you want to choose a tea based on polyphenol quality, the consensus among researchers is that green tea, which is minimally processed compared to oolong and black teas, provides the most potent polyphenols. Most of the research on tea and cancer has been conducted with green tea or green tea extracts. The National Cancer Center Research Institute in Tokyo recommends drinking green tea as one form of cancer prevention.

Green tea is now widely available in the United States, and like black tea, can be found at your local supermarket and natural food stores. Higher-quality teas can be found at tea shops. Compared to black tea, green tea is pale in color and some types can have a slightly bitter taste. If you're new to tea, flavored green teas are a great way to get into the green tea habit. Another benefit of drinking green tea is that it has half the caffeine of black tea. Remember that there are many types of tea and that taste and appearance can vary among types and brands.

If you're a black tea drinker, don't throw out your teabags yet. An eight-ounce cup of black tea still contains more antioxidants than some fruits and vegetables. Research has shown that black tea is good for the heart. (See chapter 3 for a list of health benefits.)

White tea, a very rare and expensive tea, may turn out to be the healthiest tea yet. Researchers believe that it has higher levels of the most potent polyphenols than other tea types.

Although you probably haven't heard much about rooibos tea (technically, an herbal tea), you've probably drunk it before. It's commonly used in black and herbal tea blends. Rooibos is only grown in South Africa, where it is enjoyed as a favorite beverage and valued for its healthful properties. Research in South Africa and the United States has determined that rooibos also contains antioxidant polyphenols. (See chapter 5 for more about the specific health properties of rooibos.)

ORGANIC TEAS

Another aspect to consider when selecting a tea is purity. Basically, the healthiest tea is that which undergoes the least amount of processing and moves fastest from grower to buyer. Organic teas are now more available and worth the extra cost.

Teas that are "certified organic" have been grown without the use of pesticides.

If you're looking for health benefits, avoid bottled tea drinks and powder mixes, which are generally highly processed products that are loaded with sugar and contain few, if any, polyphenols. Read labels carefully to determine nutritional content.

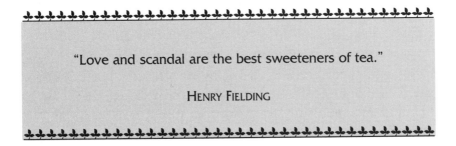

"Love and scandal are the best sweeteners of tea."

HENRY FIELDING

LOOSE OR BAGS

In terms of polyphenol content, loose and bagged teas provide the same benefits. Bags are convenient, but once you establish a tea habit, do try loose teas, which will provide you with even more varieties and flavors from which to choose.

CAFFEINE AND TEA

Tea is a natural choice if you're looking for a low-caffeine drink. As the following chart describes, black tea has half the caffeine of coffee and green tea has half the caffeine of black tea. In small amounts, caffeine in tea stimulates the central nervous system, increasing concentration and boosting energy. However, too much caffeine in the diet can cause headaches, insomnia, and other health problems.

According to the Food and Drug Administration (FDA), caffeine has been considered safe in moderation. The FDA considers 300 mg of caffeine (or seven cups of strong tea) a day to be moderate consumption. Keep in mind, though, that caffeine, like many other substances or drugs, may affect different people differently. Only you and your doctor can decide how much caffeine you can tolerate.

If you prefer to avoid caffeine, there are options. Decaffeinated tea is tea that has had the caffeine removed by a chemical process. The most common process uses ethyl acetate as a solvent, a safe procedure in terms of consumption, but not the ideal process for people who drink tea for its polyphenol content. The ethyl acetate method destroys some of the beneficial qualities of tea and wipes out 70 percent of the polyphenols.

Many health-conscious people now prefer tea that has been decaffeinated using carbon dioxide (CO_2) and water. This type of decaffeination is more expensive than ethyl acetate decaffeination, but well worth the cost because it's less damaging to tea leaves and preserves 90 percent of polyphenols. As consumers become more educated about this process, more tea companies are using CO_2 decaffeination and label their products accordingly. If you buy tea that doesn't mention which type of decaffeination process was used, you are probably safe in assuming that an ethyl acetate process was used. Whatever type of tea you buy, be aware that all decaffeinated teas contain trace amounts of caffeine.

Caffeine-free tea is tea that never contained caffeine. In other words, caffeine-free tea is made from herbs. For tea lovers who don't want to give up their morning strong black tea with milk, rooibos tea, which has a strong, rich taste similar to black tea, is a perfect alternative. It's naturally caffeine free, takes milk well, and is often organically grown. Teas made from herbs like peppermint and rosemary are reviving and stimulating but contain no caffeine. Other caffeine-free herbs like chamomile and lemon balm promote relaxation and calm the nerves. (Of the herbal teas listed in this book, only maté, also called yerba maté, contains caffeine.)

CAFFEINE CONTENT OF TEAS AND COFFEE

Beverage (8 oz)	Calories*	Caffeine**
Coffee	0	100 mg
Black tea	0	40–50 mg
Oolong tea	0	25–35 mg
Green tea	0	20–30 mg
Decaffeinated green tea	0	4 mg
Decaffeinated black tea	0	4 mg
Herbal tea	0	0 mg
Maté	0	20–150 mg
Rooibos	0	0 mg
White tea	0	20–30 mg

*Tea and coffee may have up to 3 to 4 calories per serving.
**Caffeine content will vary according to the amount of tea used and brewing times.

TEA AND IRON

You may have heard that tea interferes with the body's absorption of iron. This is true only when tea is consumed with a meal where the main source of iron comes from plants. Plant iron is less readily absorbed by the body in the presence of tea, but consuming vitamin C at the same time can increase absorption. Drinking tea during a meal containing meat will not affect the body's absorption of iron from meat sources, and drinking tea between meals has no effect on iron absorption.

MILK OR SUGAR?

Research has determined that adding milk, sugar, or lemon does not affect tea's polyphenol content or uptake of polyphenols from the gastrointestinal tract. But remember, adding milk adds calories. Once tea is brewed, you'll gain the same benefits whether you drink it hot or cold.

TEA OR SUPPLEMENTS

Now that green tea's health benefits are becoming more well known, many herbal companies are producing dietary supplements containing green tea extracts that appeal to people who don't like the taste of tea or don't have the time to prepare several cups of tea a day.

If you are interested in supplements, there are issues to consider. Since these substances are not regulated by the FDA, consumers have no real way of knowing about the quality or efficacy of supplements. Also, researchers have not yet determined if the disease-fighting substances in tea are effective alone or in combination with the other substances in the tea leaf. In other words, the general belief among scientists is that tea's polyphenols are probably more effective when consumed in their natural state.

If you do choose to use supplements, do so under the supervision of a doctor or naturopath.

YOUR DAILY CUPPAS

There's no simple prescription outlining the ideal daily tea intake. Many western studies suggest that one to two cups of tea a day can reduce heart disease risk factors. Other studies, in which subjects who drank four or five cups a day seemed to benefit more than subjects who drank one or two cups a day, indicated that perhaps when it comes to tea, more is better. Then there are the many Chinese and Japanese study results that seem to recommend that nine or ten cups of green tea a day are necessary to provide protective effects.

Japan's high green tea consumption (five to ten cups a day) may seem overwhelming to people considering adding tea to their diets. How do you have the time (or the bladder space) to drink so much in one day? And what about drinking the eight glasses of water that health professionals recommend for good health?

First, there's the matter of cup size. Teacups in Japan and China hold 60 to 100 ml (approximately two to three fluid ounces) of tea compared to larger-size western cups that hold between 170–200 ml (approximately six to seven fluid ounces) and large mugs that hold eight ounces (280 ml) or more. So the recommended ten cups of green tea a day in Japan would be about six or seven cups in Europe and North America.

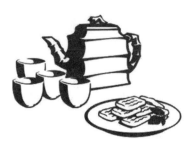

"Christopher Robin was home by this time, because it was the afternoon, and he was so glad to see them that they stayed there until very nearly tea-time, and then they had a Very Nearly tea, which is one you forget about afterwards, and hurried on to Pooh Corner, so as to see Eeyore before it was too late to have a Proper Tea with owl."

A. A. MILNE,
The House at Pooh Corner

As for your water intake, tea is mostly water, so you can substitute a few cups of tea for some of your daily water intake. Tea is also a perfect calorie-free substitute for sugary soft drinks, juices, and sports drinks, as well as caffeinated beverages. There's no need to become obsessed with tea, but you may want to increase your tea intake a bit. Many researchers agree that four to five 6- to 8-ounce cups of green or black tea a day, which is considered moderate consumption, are optimal for providing health benefits.

TEA AT EVERY MEAL

If drinking four or five cups a day seems like a lot to you, there are other ways to get your daily dose of polyphenols. Tea can be blended into breakfast smoothies, diluted and consumed after exercising, or used as a flavoring in soups, as well as meat, fish, vegetable dishes, and desserts. *Cooking With Green Tea* by Ying Chang Compestine (Avery, $16.95) is an excellent book with many wonderful recipes using green tea.

Herbal teas are another option for people who don't like the taste of tea or who simply want to try something new. While they may not contain the same types (or strength) of polyphenols, herbal teas can be refreshing and provide important healthful properties.

In the following chapter you'll read more about some of the common herbs used in teas.

5 | Treat Yourself with Tea

> *"My experience . . . convinced me that tea was better than brandy, and during the last six months in Africa I took no brandy, even when sick taking tea instead."*

THEODORE ROOSEVELT

People have been using herbs for medicinal purposes for thousands of years. Both Europe and Asia have established herbal traditions that are still practiced today alongside modern medicine. Now that herbal medicine has become more popular in this country, more people are using herbal remedies, such as herbal teas, to relieve the symptoms of common ailments like headaches, PMS, insomnia, and digestive problems.

Herbal Tea

Herbal teas, also called *tisanes*, are made from dried herbs infused in hot water, just like tea. Depending on the plant and on the ailment being treated different parts of a plant (leaves, fruit, root, flower, bark, stems, or seeds) may be infused to make tea. Some herbal teas are made using a method called decoction, where herbs (generally bark, roots, and some fruits) are boiled and left to simmer for up to an hour.

Preparing herbs as tea is an effective way to extract the water-soluble constituents in herbs that contain beneficial properties. Depending on which herbs are used, a properly prepared herbal infusion may yield anywhere from 15 to 30 percent of soluble extracts into the cup, which are more easily absorbed and utilized by the body than most powdered dried herbs in capsule form.

Teas can be made from single herbs or a combination of herbs. In Chinese and European medicine, herbs are often used in combinations to enhance their therapeutic properties.

HERBS AS MEDICINE

There are two types of herbal teas: beverage teas and medicinal teas. Many of the herbal teas sold in supermarkets in this country are beverage teas made from commercial or food-grade herbs; these teas are classified and regulated as food products. While these herbal teas are perfectly delicious drinks for all occasions, they don't contain the quality or dose of herbs necessary to be considered therapeutic.

Medicinal teas are made from higher-grade herbs. In Europe, Canada, and China, herbal teas are graded, regulated, and prescribed as pharmaceutical products. For example, in Germany, medicinal herbal teas are sold as over-the-counter drugs. Like modern medicines and over-the-counter drugs, these teas are prepared according to quality standards set by each country. The standards, established by scientists, pharmacists, doctors, and practitioners of traditional medicine (i.e., those trained in medical practices like acupuncture and herbalism that existed before modern medicine), are based on a collection of information about herbs including traditional use, scientific studies, chemical analysis, and clinical studies.

In the United States, where herbal remedies are still considered an alternative treatment, "medicinal" herbal teas are classified and regulated as dietary supplements even when they meet the quality standards for therapeutic doses of herbs as published in industry guidelines such as the *United States Pharmacopeia*, the *United States National Formulary*, and the *American Herbal Pharmacopoeia*. Many American companies producing high-quality herbal teas also consult additional herbal medicine standards such as the *European Pharmacopoeia*, the *British Herbal Pharmacopoeia*, the *German Drug Codex*, and the *German Pharmacopeia*.

GERMAN COMMISSION E

In the late 1970s Germany's Minister of Health established the German Commission E, a regulatory board that, over the following sixteen years, established guidelines for herb use. The board's primary purpose was evaluating the safety and efficacy of herbal medicines, including herbal teas, used in Germany. During this review period, herbal medicine experts (including doctors, pharmacologists, toxicologists, pharmacists, biostatisticians, non–medical health practitioners, pharmaceutical representatives, and university professors) reviewed a wide range of data on herbs, including history of traditional use, chemical analysis of herbs, pharmacological and toxicological studies, clinical studies, epidemiological studies, and medical records detailing herbal treatments. Commission E, acknowledged as the leading model for regulating the use of herbs for medicinal purposes, published its monographs (i.e., descriptions of each herb, with usage and dosage guidelines) in 1992.

In the last few years, the American Botanical Council has published two English translations of Commission E's herbal guidelines, *The Complete German Commission E Monographs— Therapeutic Guide to Herbal Medicines* and *Herbal Medicine Expanded Commission E Monographs.*

Additional organizations for which scientists continue to prepare herbal monographs include the World Health Organization (WHO) and the European Scientific Cooperative on Phytotherapy (ESCOP).

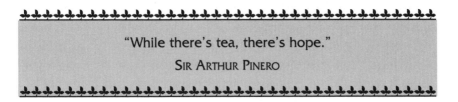

"While there's tea, there's hope."

SIR ARTHUR PINERO

SELECTING AN HERBAL TEA

With all this information about standards and efficacy, you might be wondering how to select the best quality herbal teas.

For the best results, work with a naturopath, Chinese medical doctor, herbalist, or other practitioner of traditional medicine who can prescribe an herbal tea (and a correct dosage) for your specific condition and symptoms. Some of these health professionals may prepare and sell you teas directly. Others may recommend an herbal tea brand known for its therapeutic value that can be purchased at natural food markets.

Generally, herbal teas made by companies who specialize in herbal teas and who are committed to following herbal traditions are most likely to contain high-quality herbs. The best herbal teas, from a "medicinal" standpoint, will conform to established standards regarding quality and dosage, like those published by Commission E, for medicinal use. However, it may take some time to find the highest quality teas since herbal teas are not labeled as "medicinal" in this country. If you want to learn more about the standards and quality of herbs used in a particular tea, contact the herbal tea company that makes it. Most have toll-free customer service numbers and websites.

Like black or green tea, there are many factors that influence an herbal tea's efficacy, including the quality, processing, and freshness of herbs used, and steeping time. Your health care provider or herbalist should be able to give you instructions for brewing, or refer you to the instructions on the box regarding storage and brewing. Some brands seal each teabag in a moistureproof packet to preserve freshness.

Collecting, grading, processing, and prescribing herbal remedies is a science best left to the experts. You should never collect herbs in the wild or try to make herbal remedies or teas at home because some herbs can be toxic, even deadly, if consumed or used incorrectly.

HERBS AND COMMON AILMENTS

Herbal remedies, including herbal teas, are more available and more popular with American consumers than ever before. You've probably heard about some of the top-selling herbs like echinacea, ginkgo, kava kava, ginger, St. John's wort, and ginseng. More people are turning to these natural substances to treat common conditions like PMS, anxiety, headaches, indigestion, and even mild depression.

In the following pages you'll find brief descriptions of the most important herbs, selected for their health value, efficacy, availability, and ease of use. All of these herbs are available as single herb teas or in multiherb teas that can be purchased in prepackaged teabags at grocery stores, natural food markets, and some tea specialty shops. On page 129, there is a chart that will help you select herbs by the conditions and symptoms they address.

Please note: The following descriptions of herbs are provided to help introduce you to a variety of common herbs and help you become more familiar with their uses as teas. Although herbs taken under the supervision of a doctor experienced in dispensing herbal remedies are generally very safe, some herbs may interact with prescription or over-the-counter drugs. If you have any medical conditions or concerns, discuss these with your physician before using herbal supplements or herbal teas. Some people may have sensitivities to herbs just like they might have a sensitivity to certain medications. Keep in mind that with many herbs, a small amount goes a long way.

HERBS FOR TEA

This section contains two lists of herbs used to treat common ailments. Since Commission E is considered the gold standard in evaluating herbs as medicine, I've included only herbs described in the *Herbal Medicine Expanded Commission E Monographs* in the first list. Many of these herbs are also indicated for medicinal use as teas by the German Standard License (a government organization that regulates herbal medicines in Germany). The descriptions contain information about traditional uses, followed by the approved use indicated by Commission E or the German Standard License, as described in the *Herbal Medicine Expanded Commission E Monograph*. The second list contains commonly used herbs with a tradition of folk use.

All of the herbs listed here are considered by practitioners of traditional medicine as effective treatments based on a long history of traditional use. Nearly all of the herbs listed in the monographs have also been researched in a variety of studies including in vitro, animal studies, chemical analysis, and clinical trials, in addition to their established use in traditional medicine.

Each herb's primary therapeutic use is described briefly. For specific information about supporting research, usage, dosage, contraindications, and side effects, refer to the *Herbal Medicine Expanded Commission E Monographs.* Also, consult with your physician before taking any medicine, whether it's an herbal (i.e., traditional) or modern pharmaceutical.

LIST 1: Herbs Listed in Commission E Monographs

Angelica (*Angelica archangelica*)

Traditionally, angelica has been used in Europe as an expectorant for coughs, colds, and respiratory illness and as a digestive aid. In Chinese medicine, angelica (*Angelica sinensis*), which is called dong quai, is considered the perfect all-body tonic, particularly for women. The Chinese regard dong quai as an energy tonic that strengthens the life force, or "qi" energy of the body.

A source of antioxidant vitamins B_{12} and E and magnesium, researchers believe that angelica contains high concentrations of plant chemicals that help regulate hormones, making it an ideal treatment for PMS, painful or irregular periods, and menopausal symptoms.

Angelica root tea is licensed in Germany for treating gastrointestinal and stomach ailments such as flatulence, mild cramping, and a feeling of fullness.

Tea made from: Root

Precautions: Do not use during pregnancy. Avoid prolonged exposure to sun and UV rays while using.

Bilberry (*Vaccinium myrtillus*)

Bilberry tea has been used in traditional medicine in Europe for centuries as a soothing gargle for sore throats and mouth ulcers, as well as an effective remedy for diarrhea and dysentery. Researchers suggest that bilberry may have an effect on certain eye ailments.

Bilberry tea is licensed in Germany to treat diarrhea.

Tea made from: Fruit

Chamomile, German (*Matricaria recutita*)

Highly regarded throughout history, chamomile tea has been used to soothe and calm, relieve nausea, fight bladder infections, reduce water retention, soothe body aches, and treat digestive disorders like constipation, gas, indigestion, ulcers, and cramps. The Anglo-Saxons considered it one of nine sacred herbs, and today in France chamomile tea is still one of the most consumed herbal teas.

Modern scientific studies have examined chamomile's use in topical ointments to treat skin inflammation and wounds. Although used by many people as a mild sedative and sleep aid, chamomile is not indicated for this use by Commission E due to insufficient research. Chamomile tea is licensed in Germany to treat gastrointestinal complaints and mucous membrane irritation of the mouth and throat.

Tea made from: Flower heads

Chaste Berry (*Vitex agnus castus*)

Traditionally, chaste berry was used to reduce libido. Today it's primarily used to treat a variety of menstrual problems, including breast tenderness, tension, and mood swings associated with PMS, painful periods, irregular periods, and menopausal symptoms. Researchers believe that chaste berry may contain substances that affect the pituitary gland, balancing hormone levels in women.

The German Commission E approves the use of chaste berry to treat menstrual irregularities and symptoms of PMS.

Tea made from: Berries

"Living water must be boiled with living fire,
I fetch deep clear water by the Fishing Rock
A big bucket saved the moon into a jar for spring,
A small scoop divided the stream into a bottle
for the evening."

Su Dong Po, Sung Dynasty

Dandelion (*Taraxacum officinale*)

Those pesky weeds have a purpose after all. Rich in vitamins A, B, C, D, minerals, iron, potassium, and calcium, dandelion has a variety of medicinal properties. Traditionally, dandelion was used to treat liver and spleen ailments. The Ojibwa Indians used dandelion to treat heartburn. Dandelion has been used to treat constipation, indigestion, gas, urinary tract infections, and water retention. Because it stimulates the bowels and has diuretic properties, some consider dandelion tea a diet/weight-loss aid.

In Germany, dandelion tea is licensed to treat disorders of the bile ducts/gallbladder, mild gastrointestinal problems, and to stimulate urination.

Tea made from: Leaves, roots

Dong Quai (*Angelica sinensis*). *See* Angelica.

Echinacea (*Echinacea angustifolia, purpurea, pallida*)

Used by Native Americans to treat a variety of ailments, including abscesses, boils, infected wounds, inflammation, and bug and snake bites, echinacea is now one of the best-selling herbal supplements in America and one of the most prescribed and researched in Germany. It contains potent plant chemicals that may stimulate the immune system and enhance the power of infection-fighting white blood cells. With antibacterial, antiviral, and antitumor properties, echinacea also contains B vitamins, calcium, and iron. Echinacea has been used to treat bronchitis, colds, and flu.

In Germany, *Echinacea pallida* root tea is licensed for strengthening the body's defenses against upper respiratory illnesses.

Tea made from: Root and rhizome, flower, leaf, stem

Precautions: Some researchers have posed a theoretical consideration that some uses of echinacea are not recommended for people with multiple sclerosis, lupus, or other autoimmune diseases. If you have HIV or AIDS, consult with your physician before using echinacea.

Elder (*Sambuca nigra*)

Rich in vitamin C, elder was used by Native Americans to treat headaches, reduce fevers, and clear the lungs of excess mucus. Elder continues to be used as an expectorant and decongestant in treating the symptoms of bronchitis, colds, coughing, and flu. It also increases sweating and urination to rid the body of toxins. Elder tea can be used to freshen and tone the skin, and as a gargle for sore throats.

Elder tea is licensed in Germany to increase sweating in treating fevers associated with colds and flu.

Tea made from: Flowers

Eleuthero Root (*Eleutherococcus senticosus*)

Often (incorrectly) called "Siberian ginseng" in the United States, eleuthero root is considered in China to be a restorative all-body tonic that improves health, renews energy, improves memory, increases stamina, and helps the body cope with stress. Like ginseng, eleuthero root is considered to be an adaptogen, which regulates body chemistry.

Commission E has approved the use of eleuthero root for fatigue, weakness, reduced ability to concentrate, and general impairment due to illness.

Tea made from: Root and rhizome

Precautions: Not recommended for people with hypertension, although it has been shown in some cases to reduce high blood pressure.

Fennel (*Foeniculum vulgare*)

Fennel has been used to treat gas, indigestion, inflammation and/or spasms in the digestive tract, fluid retention, constipation, and abdominal cramps. It has also been used to stimulate milk production in new mothers, reduce congestion and soothe respiratory problems like coughing and bronchitis, and to treat urinary tract infections. Some herbalists believe that fennel can be used to supplement weight-loss programs.

In Germany, fennel tea is licensed to treat flatulence, gastrointestinal tract cramping/pain, and as an expectorant for the respiratory tract.

Tea made from: Seeds

Precautions: May cause allergic reactions (respiratory and/or skin) in some people. Fennel seeds are poisonous. They must be properly processed to be used medicinally. Not recommended during pregnancy.

Fenugreek (*Trigonella-foenum-graecum*)

Ancient Egyptians, Romans, and Greeks used fenugreek to treat everything from allergies and respiratory illnesses to sore muscles, diarrhea, and fever. According to recent research, fenugreek appears to help lower blood sugar and may benefit people with type 1 or type 2 diabetes. In traditional medicine fenugreek has been used to stimulate appetite, relieve diarrhea and constipation, reduce inflammation, lower cholesterol, and soothe lungs, throat, and stomach. Commission E has approved the internal use of fenugreek to treat loss of appetite.

Tea made from: Seeds

Precautions: Drink a lot of water when using fenugreek. If you have diabetes, consult with your physician before using fenugreek. Prolonged use may cause a skin reaction. Not recommended during pregnancy.

"Tea is very, very important. The Orient discovered that thousands of years ago, and the English, having picked it up from the Orient centuries ago, perhaps overdo it a bit. But it's much too much *un*drunk in America. There's nothing healthier than tea!"

DIANA VREELAND, D.V.

Ginger (*Zingiber officinale*)

Ginger's history of use dates back to ancient China, Greece, and Rome. It has been used in traditional Asian medicine for thousands of years to treat nausea, diarrhea, and stomachaches. Loaded with potent plant chemicals, ginger is considered a warming herb that increases circulation in the body and reduces heart attack and stroke risk by lowering cholesterol levels and preventing blood clots. Ginger is also considered an excellent tonic for the digestive system; it is believed to stimulate digestion, cleanse the colon, and increase metabolism. For nausea, motion sickness, indigestion, morning sickness, or even a hangover, nothing settles the stomach like ginger tea. Ginger is also used to treat colds, flu, coughs, and chills. Research indicates that ginger might also be effective in treating inflammation and pain associated with arthritis, rheumatism, and gout.

Ginger tea is licensed in Germany to treat indigestion and to prevent motion sickness.

Tea made from: Root

Precautions: Don't take large amounts on an empty stomach. If you take blood-thinning medication or have gallstones, you should consult with your physician before taking. Not recommended during pregnancy.

Ginkgo (*Ginkgo biloba*)

At 200 million years old, ginkgo is the oldest tree species on the planet and one of the heartiest—a ginkgo tree was the only thing that survived the atomic bomb at Hiroshima. The Chinese have used ginkgo (seeds) for thousands of years to treat mental decline associated with old age and for respiratory problems like congestion and asthma. It is commonly used in blends to enhance other herbs.

Research suggests that ginkgo restores blood flow to the brain and other parts of the body, and protects brain cells from free radicals. Traditionally, it has been used to improve circulation, particularly blood flow to the brain, resulting in improved memory, concentration, vision, hearing, and balance and reduced anxiety and headaches. Scientists are examining ginkgo's potential to aid in treating Alzheimer's and sexual dysfunction.

Commission E has approved ginkgo's use for treating dizziness, memory and concentration deficiencies, headaches, tinnitus, and vascular problems in the legs.

Tea made from: Leaf and seeds

Precautions: Do not take ginkgo if you are taking monoamine oxidase inhibitors (MAOIs) for depression. If you take blood-thinning medication, you should consult with your physician before taking ginkgo as it can enhance the effects of this type of medication. Ginkgo seeds are toxic, and must be properly processed to yield therapeutic benefits.

Ginseng (*Panax ginseng*), also called Chinese Ginseng, Korean Ginseng

Ginseng has been used for medicinal purposes for at least 2000 years. It's used extensively in Chinese medicine to revitalize and restore the body's vital energy, called "qi." In the United States, ginseng is most widely known and used as a treatment for stress and fatigue. Ginseng is considered an *adaptogen,* a substance that regulates, stimulates, and balances body chemistry. Some say it can lower high blood pressure and raise low blood pressure, reduce anxiety, and tonify the body to combat the effects of stress and fatigue. Athletes have used ginseng to improve performance and heighten mental acuity. Ginseng is also considered to be an immune system enhancer that tones the thyroid and adrenal glands. Researchers are examining whether ginseng might be useful in the treatment of some types of diabetes.

Commission E indicates the use of ginseng to invigorate and fortify the body during times of fatigue and debility.

Tea made from: Root

Precautions: Do not use if you are taking a monoamine oxidase inhibitor or if you have hypertension.

Hawthorn (*Crataegus monogyna*)

Hawthorn is best known for its traditional use in treating heart disease. Research has shown that hawthorn contains powerful plant chemicals that may improve circulation and dilate and protect blood vessels in the heart, reducing the risk of atherosclerosis (clogged arteries), angina pectoris (chest pain caused by coronary disease), and high blood pressure.

At the time that the Commission E monographs were published, hawthorn had not yet been approved for therapeutic use due to insufficient research.

Tea made from: Berries, flowers, leaves

Precautions: If you have heart problems and are taking medication, consult with your physician before adding hawthorn to your regimen.

Hops (*Humulus lupulus*)

Used in beer brewing, bread making, and even as a salad topper, hops has a long tradition of therapeutic use dating back to the ninth century. Today hops is used as a mild sedative and to treat restlessness, insomnia, and indigestion in China, India, and Europe.

In Germany, hops tea is licensed to treat restlessness and sleeping disorders.

Tea made from: Strobile (flower)

Precautions: If you have depression or allergies, you should consult with your physician before using hops.

Kava Kava (*Piper methysticum*), also called Kava

If you're having trouble relaxing at the end of the day, try a cup of kava tea. Kava is considered a natural sedative and antidepressant that is used to combat anxiety, stress, and sleep-lessness.

Commission E has approved the use of kava to treat anxiety, restlessness, and stress-related conditions.

Tea made from: Root

Precautions: Do not overuse; can cause discoloration and/or scaling of the skin with prolonged use. Not recommended for persons under eighteen or during pregnancy or breast-feeding. Can enhance effects of alcohol and other drugs.

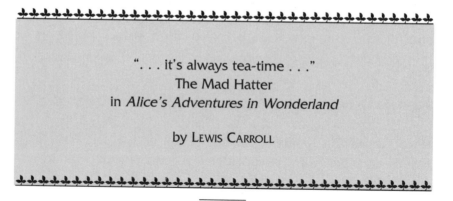

". . . it's always tea-time . . ."
The Mad Hatter
in *Alice's Adventures in Wonderland*

by Lewis Carroll

Lavender (*Lavandula angustifolia*)

Lavender has been used in traditional medicine for thousands of years. Ancient cultures used lavender as a perfume, antiseptic, and to disinfect hospital rooms. In India lavender is used to treat digestive problems and mild depression.

Lavender tea is licensed in Germany to treat nervous disorders of the stomach and intestines, restlessness, lack of appetite, and sleeplessness.

Tea made from: Flower

Lemon Balm (*Melissa officinalis*)

Antiviral and antibacterial, lemon balm was used in ancient Greece and Rome to treat wounds, bites, and stings. In India it was used to treat upset stomach caused by nervous tension or anxiety, and in the United States, it's combined with other substances to make sleep aids. Research has shown that lemon balm fights the viruses that cause mumps and herpes. In fact, in one study, a cream containing 700 mg of lemon balm was more effective at healing herpes sores than the popular drug acyclovir. Lemon balm has also been used to treat sleeplessness, gas, and indigestion.

Lemon balm tea is licensed in Germany to treat nervous disorders affecting sleep and the gastrointestinal tract and to stimulate appetite.

Tea made from: Leaves

Precautions: There is debate about whether lemon balm should be used to treat Graves' disease.

Licorice (*Glycyrrhiza glabra*)

Licorice has been widely used in traditional medicine and is the subject of extensive research. Packed with polyphenols, licorice has powerful antibacterial, antiviral, and anti-inflammatory properties. It is believed that licorice acts like a natural steroid, reducing inflammation in the lungs and stimulating adrenal function. Licorice has been used to treat coughs, sore throats, asthma, allergies, stomach irritation, and ulcers. Scientists have shown that licorice stimulates the immune system to secrete chemicals that fight viruses like Epstein-Barr, hepatitis, herpes, and HIV.

Licorice root tea is licensed in Germany to loosen phlegm in the bronchial passages in cases of bronchitis and to treat the spasms and pain associated with chronic inflammation of the gastrointestinal tract.

Tea made from: Root

Precautions: Do not take long-term; use under the supervision of a physician. Not recommended during pregnancy or for people with heart disease, high blood pressure, kidney or liver problems, or diabetes. Side effects include water retention, potassium loss, and hypertension.

Maté (*Ilex paraguayensis*), also called Yerba Maté

If you're looking for an energy boost, maté's your drink. A popular, naturally caffeinated beverage in Argentina, Brazil, and Paraguay, where it is served in a hollowed-out calabash gourd and drunk through a silver straw called a bombilla, maté has been used as a stimulant to treat mental and physical fatigue and headaches, and as a diuretic. Rich in vitamins and minerals, it's considered a nourishing all-body tonic.

Maté leaf has been approved by Commission E to treat mental and physical fatigue.

Tea made from: Leaves

Milk Thistle (*Silybum marianum*)

More than 100 studies have been conducted on milk thistle, which has been used in traditional medicine as a liver tonic, protecting the liver from toxins and free radicals.

In Germany, milk thistle tea is licensed for use to treat digestive problems and gallbladder/bile duct problems.

Tea made from: Fruit (seed)

Nettle (*Urtica dioica*), also called stinging nettle

Nettle contains antihistamines and has anti-inflammatory and diuretic properties. It has been used to treat urinary tract and prostate problems, allergies, and kidney stones, and is believed to improve circulation, fight respiratory infections, and ease the pain of inflammatory conditions like arthritis.

In Germany nettle herb tea is licensed for use to increase urination and relieve problems associated with urination.

Tea made from: Herb (leaf and flower), root (rhizomes and root)

Precautions: If you have kidney problems, consult with your physician before using nettle tea.

Parsley (*Petroselinum crispum*)

Parsley contains vitamins A, B-complex, and C, zinc, selenium, and has antioxidant and antibiotic properties. It also contains natural antihistamines. Parsley has been used for urinary tract infections, colds and coughs, allergies, and kidney stones. In Britain parsley root is used as a diuretic and to treat gas and indigestion.

Commission E has approved parsley herb and root to cleanse the urinary tract and to prevent kidney stones.

Tea made from: Leaves, root, seeds

Precautions: Do not use if you are pregnant, have kidney problems, or take monoamine oxidase inhibitors (MAOIs). May occasionally cause allergic reactions on skin and mucous membranes.

Passionflower (*Passiflora incarnata*)

Passionflower has a long history of use in traditional medicines from the Aztec Indians and Native Americans to Europeans. It has been used to treat insomnia, anxiety and nervousness, and menstrual pain.

In Germany, passionflower tea is licensed to treat restlessness, sleep disorders, and gastrointestinal complaints associated with nervous tension.

Tea made from: Aerial parts (flower, fruit, leaf)

Peppermint (*Menta piperita*)

All-purpose peppermint stimulates, enlivens, and refreshes. Traditionally, it's been used to relieve headaches, nausea, and muscle and nerve pain, and ease intestinal irritations like inflammation and irritable bowel syndrome. Peppermint is also considered a powerful decongestant that thins mucus in airways and nasal passages.

In Germany, peppermint leaf tea is licensed for treating gastrointestinal and gallbladder ailments.

Tea made from: Leaf

Precautions: If you have gallstones, consult your physician before use.

Plantain *(Plantago lanceolata)*

Plantain reduces congestion and inflammation, making it an ideal treatment for colds, coughs, allergies, and respiratory infections. Traditionally, it has been used to treat bronchitis, bladder infections, candida, colitis, itching caused by poison ivy, high blood pressure, and yeast infections. Native Americans used plantain as an antivenom for snake and spider bites. It can also be used as a gargle.

Plantain tea is licensed in Germany to reduce congestion.

Tea made from: Leaves

Precautions: Use in moderation.

Rosemary *(Rosamarinus officinalis)*

This uplifting herb stimulates the nervous system, increases circulation in the brain and throughout the body, and improves memory and concentration, refreshing mind and body. Traditionally, rosemary has been used to treat heart and circulatory conditions, indigestion, lethargy, low blood pressure, and muscle and nerve pain. Rosemary is also used as a skin and scalp toner and revitalizer.

In Germany, rosemary leaf tea is licensed to treat gastrointestinal problems like flatulence, feeling of distension, mild cramplike pain, and gallbladder/bile duct problems.

Tea made from: Leaf

Precautions: If you have epilepsy, you should consult with your physician before using. Not recommended during pregnancy.

Saw Palmetto *(Serenoa repens)*

Another top-selling herb, saw palmetto has been used to treat cystitis, stomachaches, and reproductive system disorders.

Commission E has approved the use of saw palmetto for urinary problems relating to benign prostate enlargement.

Tea made from: Berries

Senna *(Senna alexandrina)*

Senna has been used in traditional medicine (and as an ingredient in modern over-the-counter drugs) as a natural laxative to treat constipation.

In Germany, senna leaf and senna pod teas are licensed to treat constipation and as a stool softener for conditions like hemorrhoids or after surgery.

Tea made from: Leaves and pods

Precautions: Short-term use only. Do not use if you have any type of digestive, intestinal, or kidney problems. Not recommended for use during pregnancy or breast-feeding. Gastrointestinal discomfort is the primary side effect during short-term use. If you are taking diuretics, steroids, or licorice root, consult with your physician before use.

St. John's Wort *(Hypericum perforatum)*

Another top-selling herb in the United States, St. John's wort is widely used as a natural alternative to antidepressants to treat mild to moderate depression, anxiety, and insomnia. Historically, it was also used topically to treat a variety of skin conditions and wounds like burns, bruises, cuts, dermatitis, and sunburn.

St. John's wort has antibacterial, antifungal, and antiviral properties. In animal studies, scientists have discovered that St. John's wort contains a plant compound that may reduce the spread of HIV in the body. St. John's wort has been used to treat nerve pain, PMS and menopausal symptoms, incontinence, herpes, and seasonal affective disorder (SAD).

TOP-SELLING HERBS IN THE UNITED STATES

Herb	Ranking in U.S. (based on 1998 figures)
Ginkgo	1
St. John's Wort	2
Ginseng	3
Garlic	4
Echinacea/Goldenseal	5
Saw Palmetto	6
Kava Kava	7
Pycnogenol/Grape Seed	8
Cranberry	9
Valerian Root	10
Evening Primrose	11
Bilberry	12
Milk Thistle	13

Source: German Commission E

St. John's wort tea is licensed in Germany to treat sleep disturbances and nervous excitement.

Tea made from: Flowering tops (flower, bud, leaf, and stem)

Precautions: If you are taking medication for depression and/or HIV, you should consult with your physician before using St. John's wort as it may interfere with these medications. Avoid prolonged exposure to the sun while taking St. John's wort.

Thyme *(Thymus vulgares)*

Breathe easier with thyme. Antibacterial, antifungal, and antiviral, thyme contains flavonoids and other plant compounds that protect the lungs. Thyme tea has been used to soothe coughs, clear congestion and open airways, and fight viral and bacterial infections like colds, flu, and cystitis. Tea can also be used as a mouthwash or gargle for oral fungal infections.

Commission E has approved thyme for treating the symptoms of bronchitis, whooping cough, and inflammations of the upper respiratory tract and to treat some digestive problems.

Tea made from: Herb (flower and leaf)

Precautions: Not recommended during pregnancy.

"[The] three most deplorable things in the world: the spoiling of fine youths though false education, the degradation of fine paintings through vulgar admiration, and the utter waste of fine tea through incompetent manipulation."

LI CHI LAI, Sung poet

Uva Ursi *(Arctostaphylos uva ursi)*

Uva ursi, also known as bearberry, has been used for centuries by the Chinese, Europeans, and Native Americans to treat urinary tract infections.

Uva ursi tea is licensed in Germany for treating bladder and kidney inflammations.

Tea made from: Leaves

Precautions: Short-term use only. Not recommended for people with kidney problems, or for use during pregnancy, breast-feeding, or for children under the age of twelve.

Valerian *(Valeriana officinalis)*

Valerian is considered a calming and tranquilizing herb and has been used to treat anxiety, nervous tension, and insomnia.

Commission E has approved the use of valerian to treat restlessness and sleeping disorders associated with nervous conditions.

Tea made from: Root

Precautions: If you are taking medication for insomnia or depression, consult with your physician before using.

Yarrow *(Achillea millefolium)*

A multipurpose herb, yarrow has been used throughout history to treat wounds and burns. It is believed that yarrow improves digestion, stops bleeding, reduces inflammation, eliminates toxins from the blood and liver, and reduces muscle cramps and spasms.

Yarrow tea is licensed in Germany to treat spasms and cramps in the gastrointestinal tract, inflammation of the gastrointestinal tract, and to stimulate appetite.

Tea made from: Flowering tops (flower, leaf, and stem)

Precautions: Some people may be allergic to yarrow. Not recommended during pregnancy.

LIST 2: Herbs Used in Folk Remedies

(Therapeutic claims for these herbs have not been approved by Commission E. Descriptions are based on folk remedies.)

Alfalfa *(Medicago sativa)*

A rich source of minerals (iron, calcium, manganese, potassium, and phosphorus), alfalfa also contains vitamins A, D, E, G, and K. Originally used as horse and cattle feed, alfalfa, in the form of sprouts, is now used as a salad topper. Alfalfa tea may help control blood sugar levels in people with diabetes and may help lower cholesterol. It has also been used to stimulate appetite, aid in digestion, combat symptoms of menopause, and reduce water retention.

Tea made from: Leaves

Precautions: Use in small amounts. Do not use if you have an autoimmune disorder (e.g., lupus).

Astragalus *(Astragalus membranaceous),* called Huang Qi in China

Indigenous to China, astragalus is considered by some to be a powerful immune system booster that protects the body against environmental factors and augments the healing properties of other herbs. With antibacterial, anti-inflammatory, and antiviral properties, astragalus has been used to fight colds, lower blood pressure, restore adrenal function, lower high blood sugar, increase urine output in the kidneys, and stimulate the production of the body's natural antibodies to fight disease.

Tea made from: Root

Cranberry *(Vaccinium macrocarpon, Vaccinium oxycoccos)*

Cranberry tea is considered a remedy for urinary tract infections (UTIs). An effective antiseptic, cranberry prevents *E. coli* (the primary cause of most UTIs) from clinging to bladder walls and fights other bacteria that cause bladder and kidney infections. Cranberry has also been used to treat water retention. In order to get an efficacious dose of cranberry in a teabag some herbal tea companies add a dried juice concentrate to their tea.

Tea made from: Berries

Cramp Bark *(Viburnum opulus)*

Anti-inflammatory, antispasmodic, and astringent, cramp bark tea is considered an ideal tonic for women who suffer from PMS and/or painful periods. Cramp bark has been used to relieve uterine, back, and leg pain, abdominal cramps, and bloating associated with menstruation.

Tea made from: Bark

Feverfew *(Chrysanthemum parthenium, Tanacetum parthenium)*

Traditionally feverfew was used to reduce fevers. Today, researchers are studying its potential to treat migraines.

Tea made from: Leaves, flowers, stems

Precautions: Not recommended for people taking blood-thinning medications.

Goldenseal *(Hydrastis canadensis)*

With its antibiotic, antiseptic, anti-inflammatory, antifungal, antiviral, and antiparasitic properties, goldenseal was used by Native Americans to treat a wide range of ailments. Goldenseal has been used to treat eye, respiratory, parasitic, urinary tract, and vaginal infections, as well as menstrual problems and skin conditions and wounds. Goldenseal tea can be used as a gargle for mouth infections and sore throats.

Tea made from: Root and rhizome

Precautions: Short-term use only; use under the supervision of your physician.

Gotu Kola *(Centella asiatica)*

Gotu kola has been used in Ayurvedic medicine to rejuvenate mind and body. It may be helpful in healing skin and tissue wounds and improving symptoms in people with varicose veins and other vein disorders. Some consider gotu kola a brain tonic that may improve circulation in the brain, promote mental clarity, and improve concentration and memory. Elephants, known for their long lives and excellent memories, eat gotu kola leaves.

Tea made from: Herb (dried aerial parts)

Precautions: If you are being treated for depression, high blood pressure, or high cholesterol, consult with your physician before using gotu kola.

Hibiscus

A rich source of vitamin C and iron, hibiscus is considered a calming herb, and is often added to herbal blends. A recent human clinical trial showed that drinking hibiscus tea significantly lowered blood pressure, confirming earlier results from in vitro studies.

Tea made from: Flowers

Hyssop *(Hyssopus officinalis)*

Hyssop tea has been used to relieve a variety of respiratory problems. It is believed to break up congestion and phlegm in the lungs, soothe and cleanse inflamed mucous membranes, and clear airways. Hyssop has also been use to treat inflamed joints.

Tea made from: Flowers, leaves, stems

Papaya *(Carica papaya)*

Papaya has been used to treat digestive ailments like heartburn and indigestion. It also contains a protein that some believe may help thin the blood, preventing blood clots.

Tea made from: Fruit, juice, leaves, seeds

Pau d'Arco *(Tabebuia impetiginosa)*

Pau d'Arco is believed to fight bacterial, viral, and fungal infections and boost the body's immune system. It has been used to treat fungal infections, including candida, eczema, psoriasis, and vaginal yeast infections.

Tea made from: Inner bark

Raspberry *(Rubus idaeus)*

Most commonly used for intestinal and menstrual ailments, raspberry tea may treat diarrhea, reduce pain from menstrual cramps, and fight viruses and fungus. Some researchers believe that raspberry can relax the muscles of the uterus during pregnancy. Raspberry tea can also be used as a mouthwash or gargle to treat sores and inflammation in the mouth.

Tea made from: Leaf

Rooibos *(Aspalathus linearis),* also spelled Rooibosch

Grown in South Africa, rooibos tea is a caffeine-free drink that South Africans believe has many important health benefits. It contains calcium, potassium, magnesium, zinc, and sodium, and many trace elements, including fluoride and copper. Rooibos also contains flavonoids that scientists believe may function as antioxidants. Traditional uses of rooibos tea include treatment of nausea, vomiting, heartburn, constipation, stomach cramps, colic in infants, allergies (including hayfever, asthma, and eczema), and skin irritations.

Tea made from: Leaf

COMMON AILMENTS AND HEALING HERBS

Common Ailments, Symptoms, and Concerns	Healing Herbs*
Allergies	Elder, Feverfew, Ginkgo, Hyssop, Lemon Balm, Milk Thistle, Parsley, Thyme
Anxiety	Hops, Kava Kava, Lemon Balm, Passionflower, Rosemary, St. John's Wort
Arthritis	Alfalfa + Peppermint, Chamomile, Cinnamon, Dong Quai, Feverfew, Ginger, Nettle
Asthma	Feverfew, Gingko, Green Tea, Hyssop, Lemon Balm, Nettle, Parsley, Plantain, Thyme
Bladder infection	Chamomile, Cranberry
Blood pressure, high	Ginger, Ginseng, Green Tea, Hawthorn
Cholesterol, high	Ginger, Ginseng, Green Tea
Cold	Echinacea, Elder, Ginger + Peppermint, Goldenseal, Lemon, Plantain
Constipation	Dandelion, Fennel, Papaya, Senna

Common Ailments, Symptoms, and Concerns	Healing Herbs*
Cough	Elder, Peppermint, Wild Cherry
Depression	Ginseng, Lavender Flower, Lemon Balm, St. John's Wort
Digestion	Peppermint, Fennel, Fenugreek, Hops, Papaya, Yarrow, Ginger, Anise Seed, Caraway Seed, Chamomile Flower
Energy	Ginseng
Fatigue	Astragalus, Ginseng, Milk Thistle, Pau d'Arco, Rose Hips, Saw Palmetto, Maté
Fever	Echinacea, Elder Flower, Lemon, Yarrow
Flu	Echinacea, Elder, Lemon Balm, Thyme
Gas	Cinnamon, Fennel, Papaya, Peppermint
Headache	Feverfew, Ginkgo, Lavender, Parsley, Peppermint, Rosemary
Insomnia	Chamomile, Hops, Lemon Balm, Licorice, Passionflower, Valerian
Laxative	Senna
Mental clarity	Ginkgo
Muscle aches	Chamomile, Cramp Bark, Hyssop, St. John's Wort
Nausea	Ginger, Peppermint

Treat Yourself with Tea

Common Ailments, Symptoms, and Concerns	Healing Herbs*
Nervousness	Damiana, Hops, Lavender, Peppermint, Rosemary, St. John's Wort
PMS	Chaste Berry, Dong Quai, Hops, Raspberry
Sleep	Chamomile, Hops, Passionflower, Valerian
Sore Throat	Bilberry, Elder, Thyme, Echinacea Root, Licorice, Marshmallow Leaf, Marshmallow Root, Slippery Elm Bark
Stress	Ginseng, Kava Kava, Licorice, Peppermint, Maté
Tension (nervous tension)	Lavender Flower, Lemon Balm, Hops, Kava Kava, Passionflower, Valerian
Weight Control/Loss	Alfalfa, Dandelion, Ginger, Green Tea, Papaya, Birch Leaf, Dandelion Herb, Fennel, Nettle, Tea Leaf (green or black), Uva Ursi

*Not all herbs listed in this chart are described in this book.

MAKING HERBAL TEA

The simplest way to make herbal teas is to use prepackaged herbal teabags. Or, your herbalist might prepare herbs in muslin teabags for you. Generally, you use one teaspoon of herbs per cup.

When making herbal teas, follow the basic tea infusion procedure described on page 141. Use the best quality water you can. Place the tea in the cup. Add hot water (just off of boiling) to the cup and let the tea steep for 10 to 15 minutes. Cover the teacup during steeping to retain heat. Different teas will require different steeping times and methods, so follow the instructions on the tea box or from your herbalist.

You'll notice that herbal teas are generally infused longer than black or green tea. The longer steeping time is needed for the hot water to break down the cell walls of the dried herbs, releasing the beneficial substances. Sometimes dried herbal extracts are added to herbal teabags because they provide the herb's beneficial substances without requiring a longer steeping time.

6 Buying, Storing, and Brewing Tea

"Tea is nought but this; first you heat the water, then you make the tea. Then you drink it properly. That is all you need to know."

SEN RIKYU

Finally, it's teatime, a simple pleasure enjoyed morning, afternoon, and evening. Whether you take your tea in solitude or with friends, as a morning stimulant or relaxing bedtime brew, there are a few simple guidelines that will help you prepare the perfect cup of tea.

DISCOVER TEA

As you read in chapter 4, visiting a specialty tea shop with a knowledgeable staff is an excellent way to learn more about tea. Most important, you'll be able to sample tea that has been brewed correctly. You'll also be able to ask questions about the different types of tea. In addition to the five main categories of tea, there are different grades of tea based on tea leaf characteristics.

TEA GRADES

Grading systems are used by growers, primarily in India, Ceylon, and China to classify tea by leaf size and appearance, and sometimes also by rolling method. While there are many different tea grades, there is no universal grading system, so teas from these countries might be graded according to different criteria.

> "The way of tea cannot be taught in any book . . .
> it is a state of mind. Tea is a living tradition."
>
> PROFESSOR KIMIKO GUNJI, University of Illinois

Basically, tea leaves are classified into two grades, whole leaf or broken. Whole leaf tea grades are, in descending order, Orange Pekoe (whole leaf), Pekoe (smaller whole leaves), and Souchong (broad whole leaves). Broken leaf tea grades include Broken Orange Pekoe, Broken Pekoe, and Broken Pekoe Souchong, Fannings, and Dust (the smallest tea leaf particles, used in teabags). "Tippy" and "flowery" grades, which indicate the presences of intact leaf/bud tips in the tea, are generally used only to describe Indian or Ceylon teas. Some of these grades in-

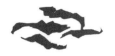  

clude Flowery Orange Pekoe, Golden Flowery Orange Pekoe, Tippy Golden Flowery Orange Pekoe.

You've probably seen the name "Orange Pekoe" (pekoe sounds like peck-o) or the initials "OP" on tea packages. The orange in orange pekoe does not refer to the fruit but was originally used by Dutch traders to suggest a link between their tea and the royal family, the House of Orange. The word "Pekoe," derived from "Pak-ho," the Chinese word that describes a baby's fine white hair, refers to the white downy tea leaf buds. The name orange pekoe is used to categorize whole leaf tea from India and Ceylon.

However, some tea companies incorrectly label black tea (particularly bagged tea) as orange pekoe to indicate taste quality when the term actually refers to tea leaf size (i.e., whole leaf tea). Teabags are made from the smallest tea particles, called dust.

Green teas are classified by plucking and rolling methods. The finest green teas are made from the bud and first leaf; following in descending order are teas made from the bud and first two leaves, then the bud and first three leaves, and so on. (See plucking diagram on page 5.)

This grading system can seem very confusing. Don't worry

about memorizing it, just remember that there are many ways of classifying tea. Basically, look for taste. The charts in chapter 1 should give you an idea of some taste characteristics of well-known teas; go ahead and try them all!

WHOLE LEAF VS. TEABAGS

With the exception of tea connoisseurs, who drink only the finest teas, most tea drinkers in this country drink black tea made from teabags. (Teabags contain the smallest tea particles left over from processing called "dust.") Some tea experts may scoff at teabags as inferior tea—their palates are developed enough to distinguish the slightest nuances between premium teas—but there are several benefits of using bagged tea. It tastes great and it's inexpensive, convenient for busy people, portable, easy to prepare at home or at work, and provides the same health benefits as whole leaf teas. Remember, if it tastes good to you, it's a good tea.

However, if you've never tried whole leaf tea before it's worth buying a bag to experience the magic of tea leaves coming to life before your eyes. (The moment the hot water hits the leaves and they begin to twist and unfurl in the water is called "the agony of the leaves.") Green teas are especially captivating to watch. One or two minutes after adding water, the cup is filled with whole tea leaves, standing on end, waving and dancing like seaweed at the bottom of the ocean.

WHERE TO BUY TEA

Bagged and loose leaf teas can be purchased at tea shops, supermarkets, and natural food stores. There are also several mail-order companies that sell premium teas. Black tea is widely available in supermarkets, and green tea is becoming more available. Basically, you can't go wrong with some of the well-known brands of black teas if you're looking for a strong, black breakfast tea. Only specialty tea shops sell the rarer white and pu'erh teas, as well as the premium whole leaf teas.

In general, when buying tea at a tea shop, price will be an indicator of quality, although inexperienced tea drinkers might not be able to tell the difference between good tea and premium teas. If you do appreciate premium teas, they are worth the extra cost. For example, even a tea that costs $100 a pound will make 200 cups of tea. That's only fifty cents per cup, a very affordable luxury. Another place to look for tea is at ethnic grocery stores. Chinese, Southeast Asian, and Indian markets often sell wonderful quality teas from their native countries.

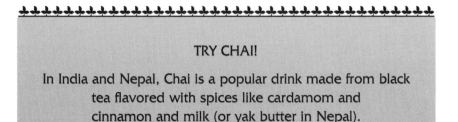

TRY CHAI!

In India and Nepal, Chai is a popular drink made from black tea flavored with spices like cardamom and cinnamon and milk (or yak butter in Nepal).

STORING TEA

Unlike fine wines, tea does not improve with age. (One exception is the smoked, aged pu'erh tea.) For this reason, it's wise to buy a small amount of tea and store it properly to preserve freshness.

In Japan, where dedicated tea drinkers seek out the freshest teas, vendors often heavily discount or throw out green tea that's more than a week old. However, any tea you buy in this country will have already been stored for packing and shipping. Tea has a fairly low moisture content, so if stored properly it can stay fresh from several weeks up to a year.

Here are a few guidelines for storing tea:

- Store tea in an airtight container. Metal, ceramic, and even wooden containers with tight-fitting lids are ideal. Some teabags come sealed in foil to preserve freshness.
- Store tea in a cool, dark place away from heat and light.
- Store only tea in your containers to avoid other substances altering the flavor of your tea.
- You may want to have separate containers for black, green, and herbal teas. Scented teas should also be stored separately.
- Buy tea in small quantities so that you can store it properly and use it up before it gets old and loses flavor. Most experts recommend using tea within six months for best taste.

Others believe that a well-preserved tea can last for up to a year before quality suffers. Green tea loses quality faster than black tea. (Freshness may also depend on how well the tea has been stored from plantation to dealers to retailers.)

Brewing Tea

Before you begin the brewing process, find out how many cups of tea your teapot can hold by measuring out cups of water and pouring them into the teapot. (The typical rounded ceramic British teapot holds a bit more than five cups of water.) This will help you know how much tea to use. For your enjoyment, use the best tea you can afford.

Although brewing tea is a simple procedure, there will be slight variations for different types of tea. Below are the basic procedures for infusing tea:

"Thank God for tea! What would the world do without tea!
How did it exist? I am glad I was not born before tea."

REV. SIDNEY SMITH

1. Fill a teakettle or saucepan with freshly drawn cold water.
   As ancient tea masters have said, the quality of water used influences the quality of the tea produced. Use filtered or bottled springwater if available.

2. For black and rooibos teas, bring the water to a boil, and for oolongs, a bit less than a full boil. If you are making green or herbal tea, stop short of boiling. Boiling water can damage delicate green tea leaves and result in a bitter-tasting tea.
   The correct boiling temperature for most black teas is around 212° F, 190–200° F for

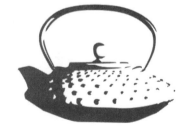

oolongs, and between 170–185° F for green teas. If you don't want to use a thermometer, you can learn to read the water instead.

Here are some visual guidelines to help you understand the different boiling times: When small bubbles begin forming on the bottom of the pan, take the water off the burner if you're making green or herbal teas. When those small bubbles begin rising to the surface (but don't break the surface of the water), the water is ready for oolong teas. For black and rooibos teas, and some oolong teas, take the pan off the burner as soon as the water begins to boil (i.e., bubbles rise to the top and break the surface of the water). If you have extra water in the pan after making tea, it's okay to reuse that water the next time you make tea. However, water should not be reboiled more than four times.

3. Pour a small amount of boiling water into the teapot and swirl it around to warm the teapot. Then empty the teapot.

4. Add one teabag or one teaspoon of tea (or herbs) to your teapot for each cup of tea you'll be serving. Or, if you're making one cup of tea, place one teabag or one teaspoon of herbs or tea in the cup.

Some people add an extra teabag or teaspoon of tea, "for the pot," but if you're using quality tea you shouldn't have to do that. As you become more experienced in making tea, you may find that you like your tea stronger or weaker.

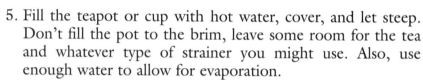

5. Fill the teapot or cup with hot water, cover, and let steep. Don't fill the pot to the brim, leave some room for the tea and whatever type of strainer you might use. Also, use enough water to allow for evaporation.

   General steeping guidelines are as follows: For black, oolong, and rooibos teas, steep between 4 and 6 minutes. For green teas, steep 1 to 3 minutes. White teas, up to 2 minutes. Herbal teas are generally steeped longer, for 10 to 15 minutes.

   Steeping times will vary. If you buy your tea from a tea shop, make sure that you ask for brewing instructions. Most tea shops will attach instructions to your bag of tea. Prepackaged teas will come with brewing and steeping instructions.

6. For iced tea, brew as normal. After tea has cooled, store in refrigerator or add ice.

7. Clean your teapot when you're through. If you use a ceramic pot, rinsing with water is enough. If you're using an iron Japanese pot, rinse and pat dry with a towel.

A FEW TIPS ON STEEPING

- Whole leaf tea requires a longer steeping time than tea made from teabags.
- For stronger tea, steep longer (not recommended for green, white, pu'erh teas).
- For a lower caffeine content (in black tea), shorten brewing time.
- Smaller tea particles, like dust in teabags, release more caffeine than whole leaf teas in the same brewing time.

UTENSILS

Although Lu Yu mentions twenty-four essential utensils in his book of tea (*Ch'A Ching*), you really only need a few implements.

First, you need something in which to boil the water. To start, just use a saucepan to boil water. It's cheaper than a kettle, and you'll be able to watch the water as it boils, becoming more familiar with boiling temperatures. Save the money you'd spend on a fancy kettle for fancy tea instead.

Some tea experts recommend having separate teapots for green, black, and scented teas, but if you use a ceramic pot and rinse it well with water after each use, you should be fine. Or, you can make tea by the cup.

For whole and other loose leaf teas, you'll need some type of straining device for infusion. One method is to make the tea in the pot and, as you pour the tea into each cup, place a small mesh strainer over it to catch tea leaves. These strainers, made from metal or bamboo, cost approximately two to four dollars.

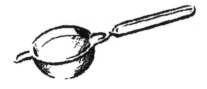

Some tea experts recommend metal utensils because they believe that bamboo can influence the taste of the tea. Others warn against aluminum utensils, which can turn tea black. In general, tea balls (cup or pot size) are not ideal for whole leaf teas because they don't allow enough room for the tea to expand.

When straining tea, it's best to remove the tea from the water rather than the water from the tea. The best strainers are gold-plated infuser cups that can be placed in the teapot or in a cup and removed after steeping. Ceramic teacups with removable strainers and lids are also ideal for making tea by the cup. T-Sacs, large paper mesh pouches that resemble empty teabags, can also be used for straining. They are available in cup and teapot sizes.

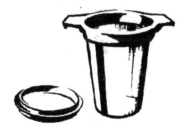

INFUSIONS

Generally, a single portion—either cup or pot size—of black tea leaves is infused only once. High-quality oolong and pu'erh teas can often be infused from the same leaves several times. Some green teas, which only require infusion times of one minute or less, can also be used more than once.

> "'Do you want your adventure now,' Peter said casually to John, 'or would you like to have your tea first?' Wendy said, 'Tea first, quickly.'"
>
> J. M. BARRIE, *Peter Pan*, 1904

DECAFFEINATING YOUR TEA

If you want to "decaffeinate" your tea, steep for thirty seconds and then pour off the water. Immediately infuse the same tea leaves with more hot water and steep for the time required for your particular tea type. Because most of the tea's caffeine is released within twenty to thirty seconds of steeping time, this method will help you reduce the caffeine content of your tea while preserving the tea's beneficial qualities and taste.

SERVING

Serving tea can be an elaborate and lengthy ritual, a simple gesture of hospitality, or a calming moment of solitude. If you're having a tea party, get out the fine china and your best silver and serve black tea with milk, sugar, and plenty of scones and other treats. Or maybe you prefer a stylized Japanese ceremony with strong matcha and a light snack. Whether you have a big tea party or enjoy your tea alone, you'll need to know how to serve the different types of tea. Some teas go well with milk, others are best consumed plain.

Here is a breakdown of some types of tea and how they are commonly served.

- In general, black teas and tea blends from Ceylon and India can be served with a bit of cold milk, and sometimes with sugar. Included in this group are Irish and English breakfast teas, which are always served with milk. Some black teas are suggested as morning teas, some as afternoon teas, and others as evening teas. Generally milk is only used in the morning (except for in Britain, where milk is always added to black tea).

- South African rooibos tea can be drunk black or with milk. It doesn't need sugar, but some people like to drink it sweetened with honey or lemon. Rooibos also blends well with soy milk (rooibos with vanilla soy milk is a perfect blend of sweet and strong flavors).

- Nothing is added to green, white, and oolong teas from China and Japan, or to most Darjeeling teas.

- China's black teas are often stronger than Ceylon and India teas, and are often served with milk or sugar.

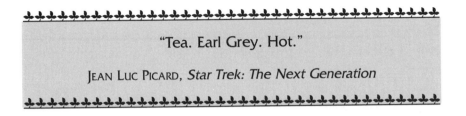

"Tea. Earl Grey. Hot."

JEAN LUC PICARD, *Star Trek: The Next Generation*

OTHER USES OF TEA

Tea isn't just a refreshing beverage; it contains vitamins, minerals, antioxidants, and other properties that make it useful around the house, too. Spent tea leaves can be added to composting piles and used to clean, deodorize, and disinfect garbage disposals.

Asian women have included green tea in their daily grooming rituals as a skin cleanser and toner for centuries. Adding a few heaping teaspoons of scented or herbal tea to your bathwater is an easy way to enjoy tea's soothing and aromatic qualities. Tea can also be used as an astringent to clean minor cuts and bug bites and as a compress to soothe and relieve the pain of sunburn or itchy skin caused by allergies. Many people swear by used teabags to reduce puffiness around the eyes. Teabags can be stored in the refrigerator and placed on closed eyes for ten to fifteen minutes while you lie down for a nap.

"I learned to take delight in the pleasure afforded by a cup of tea. When I would go in at dusk, the gentle warmth of tea filled me as night closed in around my eyrie. A simple cup of tea has often been the only spark needed to make an acquaintance, inaugurating a bond of friendships that could last a lifetime!"

P. BRUNETON, *En solitaire dans l'Himalaya*

Today many cosmetic companies are using green tea and green tea extracts in all types of skin, hair, and beauty products like soaps, lotions, perfumes, facial cleansers and lotions, shampoos, and deodorants.

One of the most well-known therapeutic uses for tea is recommended by podiatrists—tea foot baths. The tannic acid in black tea fights bacteria and closes pores. If you have stinky, sweaty feet, try this foot soak from *The Little Foot Care Book*:

Make a pint of tea using two teabags. Boil the water for fifteen minutes (with teabags in the water). Add tea to two quarts of cold water. Soak feet in cooled solution for thirty minutes. Try this foot soak every day for a week to keep your feet dryer and better smelling.

THE VIRTUES OF TEA

Our taste for tea knows no bounds. Cultures around the world have enjoyed tea's soothing and refreshing qualities for thousands of years. From the time it was discovered tea has been valued as much for its healthful properties as for its exotic flavors and aromas. No other beverage is available in so many varieties, has so many uses, and is enjoyed by people of all ages and walks of life.

Throughout history, tea has inspired writers, poets, spiritual leaders, and statesmen. British writer William Cowper called tea "the cup that cheers but not inebriates," and Samuel Johnson's addiction to tea was legendary. For some, like Chinese poet T'ien Yiheng "tea is drunk to forget the din of the world." And still for others tea and the art of preparing and serving it became codified as a spiritual practice, and even a way of life. Okakura Kakuzo (1862–1913), author of *The Book of Tea* wrote, "The tea ceremony is more than an idealization of the form of drinking—it is a religion of the art of life."

Tea has become such a part of our daily lives and collective consciousness that everyone seems to have a favorite tea, and every culture its favorite tea-drinking occasions and rituals. Our attraction to tea goes way beyond the simple beverage or its taste. The transcendence comes from experiencing tea—preparing the leaves, sharing a cup with friends, slowing down.

As you discover your own "way of tea," may you enjoy tranquillity, health, and happiness.

7 | Teasources

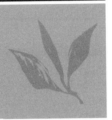

Here are some of the teas and tea products that I've sampled.

Tea Companies in U.S., U.K., South Africa

Good Earth
831 Almar Ave.
Santa Cruz, CA 95060
831-423-7913
www.goodearthteas.com

Bigelow
201 Black Rock Turnpike
Fairfield, CT 06432
800-562-5933
www.bigelowtea.com

Celestial Seasonings
4600 Sleepytime Dr.
Boulder, CO 80301-3292
www.celestialseasonings.com
800-351-8175

Twinings
216 The Strand
London, England
United Kingdom
www.twinings.com

Dragonfly
PO Box 125
Newbury, Berkshire
RG20 9FY United Kingdom
+44 (0) 16325 278648
www.dragonfly-teas.com

Eleven O'Clock
PO Box 125
Newbury, Berkshire
RG20 9FY United Kingdom
+44 (0) 16325 278648
www.rooiboschtea.com

Dilmah Tea
PO Box 1630
Columbo 10, Sri Lanka
+(94) 1 933070
www.dilmahtea.com

Five Roses
John Sommer, Inc.
24 Digital Dr., Suite 4
Novato, CA 94949
800-422-2595
www.five-roses.com

Lipton
800 Sylvan Ave.
Englewood Cliffs, NJ 07632
1-888-547-8668
www.liptont.com

Republic of Tea
8 Digital Dr., Suite 100
Novato, CA 94949
800-298-4832
www.republicoftea.com

Stash
PO Box 910
Portland, OR 97207
800-547-1514
www.stashtea.com

Taylors of Harrogate
Pagoda House
Prospect Rd.
Harrogate HG2 7NX
United Kingdom
+44 (0) 1423 889822

Sportea
7340 S. Alton Way, Unit K
Englewood, CO 80112
303-694-6965

Whittards of Chelsea
Union Court
22 Union Rd.
London, England SW4 6JQ
United Kingdom
www.whittard.com

Tetley GB Limited
325 Oldfield Ln. North
Greenford Middlesex
  UB6 0AZ
United Kingdom
0800-387-227
www.teafolk.com

Tetley USA, Inc.
100 Commerce Dr.
PO Box 856
Shelton, CT 06484-0856
800-728-0084
www.tetleyusa.com

Yogi Tea
Golden Temple of Oregon, Inc.
2545 Prairie Rd.
Eugene, OR 97402
800-yogi-tea
800-359-2940
www.yogitea.com

Companies specializing in "therapeutic" herbal teas

Alvita
A Twinlab Division
American Fork, UT 84003

Traditional Medicinals
4515 Ross Rd.
Sebastopol, CA 95472
800-373-3832
www.traditionalmedicinals.com

Good Earth Medicinals
831 Almar Ave.
Santa Cruz, CA 95060
831-423-7913
www.goodearthteas.com

Tea shops/mail order

Tea Cup
2207 Queen Anne Ave.
 North
Seattle,WA 98109
206-283-5931
www.tearanch.com

TeaSource
752 Cleveland Ave. South
St. Paul, MN 55116
877-768-7233
www.teasource.com

Upton Tea Imports
231 South St.
Hopkinton, MA 01748
800-234-8327
www.uptontea.com

Todd & Holland
7577 Lake St.
River Forest, IL 60305
800-747-8827
www.todd-holland.com

Specialteas
2 Reynolds St.
Norwalk, CT 06855-1015
888-365-6983
www.specialteas.com

TenRen
380 Swift Ave., Suite 5
South San Francisco,
 CA 94080
650-583-1044
www.tenren.com

Tea in beauty products

Pure & Basic
20600 Belshaw Ave.
Carson, CA 90746
800-432-3787
www.pureandbasic.com

Aubrey Organics
4419 N. Manhattan Ave.
Tampa, FL 33614
800-237-4270
www.aubrey-organics.com

Abra Therapeutics, Inc.
10365 Highway 16
Forestville, CA 95436
800-745-0761
www.abratherapeutics.com

Jason Natural Cosmetics
Culver City, CA 90232-2484
877-jason-05
www.jason-natural.com

The Thymes
420 N. Fifth St., Suite 1100
Minneapolis, MN 55401
800-366-4071
www.thymes.com

Tea in cleaning products

Caldrea
420 N. Fifth St., Suite 1030
Minneapolis, MN 55401
612-371-0003

Tea information

Tea Council of the USA
Tea Association of USA, Inc.
420 Lexington Ave.
New York, NY 10170
212-986-9415
www.teausa.com/
  council.html
www.teausa.com/
  association.html

The Tea Council Ltd.
9 The Courtyard
Gowan Ave.
Fulham, London SW66RH
England
United Kingdom
020 7371 7787
www.teacouncil.co.uk

**American Premium Tea
  Institute**
www.teainstitute.org

8 | Glossary

Amino Acids
The building blocks of proteins. Of the twenty amino acids essential to health, eleven occur naturally in the body. The remaining nine must be supplied by diet.

Antioxidant
A substance present in the body and in foods that protects the body against free radicals, unstable oxygen molecules that damage cells and tissues. Scientists believe that damage from free radicals contributes to illness, heart disease,

and cancer. For this reason, scientists recommend a diet rich in foods containing antioxidants. (See "Free Radical.")

Atherosclerosis

Hardening of the arteries. Occurs when fatty deposits in the arteries block blood flow.

Caffeine

A chemical found in tea that acts as a stimulant.

Carcinogen

Any cancer-causing agent.

Catechin

A type of polyphenol found in tea. Catechins are a type of flavonoid and function as antioxidants.

Chanoyu

Japanese tea ceremony.

Cholesterol

A fat-soluble substance naturally produced in liver that is used in the body's metabolism. Cholesterol is also found in animal products. High levels of cholesterol in the body are associated with an increased risk of heart attack and heart disease. Cholesterol levels are determined by the ratio of two types of cholesterol, HDL and LDL. (See "HDL," "LDL.")

DNA

Deoxyribonucleic acid. A substance found in all of the body's cells that contain an individual's genetic code.

Flavonoid

A type of polyphenol found in tea.

Free Radical

A highly reactive, unstable oxygen molecule that causes damage to the body's cells and tissues. This process occurs naturally, but exposure to toxins through air pollution, smoking, poor diet, and other stresses, can also contribute to free radical activity.

HDL

High-density lipoprotein. Often referred to as the "good" cholesterol because it helps reduce and eliminate excess cholesterol in the bloodstream.

Hypertension

High blood pressure.

In vitro

"In glass." In vitro studies are conducted by mixing substances in test tubes or other containers to determine how these substances interact with one another.

In vivo

Studies conducted using live subjects, either animals or humans. Subjects are exposed to substances to determine how these substances impact their health.

LDL

Low-density lipoprotein. Often referred to as the "bad" cholesterol because it leaves cholesterol deposits in the bloodstream, increasing heart disease risk.

Metastasis

The spread of cancerous cells. When a cancer metastasizes, it moves to another part of the body.

Oxidation

When an atom or molecule loses one or more electrons. Sometimes this process creates an unstable molecule that reacts with other molecules, causing cell damage.

Phytochemicals

Plant chemicals that scientists believe play a role in protecting the body from disease and illness.

Polyphenols   A type of plant chemical (i.e., phytochemical) found in foods like grapes and onions, and in tea. Some polyphenols function as antioxidants. (See "Flavonoid," "Catechin.")

Rhizome   A rootlike, lateral plant stem that grows underground and sends out roots from its lower surface.

Tannins   A type of flavonoid in tea that has antioxidant properties. Tannins give tea its taste and color.

Notes

Sources consulted during research include interviews with leading tea researchers and with tea and herb experts, books, press kits, and fact sheets provided by tea companies, print and online articles, and websites and printed materials provided by non-profit national tea councils.

Books

Blofeld, J., *The Chinese Art of Tea* (Boston: Shambala, 1985).

Blumenthal, M., Goldberg, A., and Brinckmann, J., *Herbal Medicine Expanded Commission E Monographs* (Newton, MA: Integrative Medicine Communications, 2000).

Burgess, A., *The Book of Tea* (Paris: Flammarian, 1992).

Duke, J. A., *The Green Pharmacy Herbal Handbook* (Emmaus, PA: Rodale, 2000).

Griffith, H. W., *Healing Herbs* (Tucson: Fisher Books, 2000).

Gustafson, H., *The Agony of the Leaves* (New York: Henry Holt and Company, 1996).

Hall, D., *The Herb Tea Book* (New Canaan, CT: Keats Publishing, Inc., 1981).

Kakuzo, O., *The Book of Tea* (Boston: Tuttle Publishing, 2000).

Manchester, C., *Tea in the East* (New York: Hearst Books, 1996).

Mitscher, L., Dolby, V., *The Green Tea Book* (New York: Avery Publishing Group, 1998).

Murray, M. T., *The Healing Power of Herbs* (Rocklin, CA: Prima Publishing, 1995).

NOTES

Norman, J., *Teas and Tisanes* (London: Dorling Kindersley, 1989).

Norwood Pratt, J., *The Tea Lover's Companion* (New York: Carol Publishing Group, 1996).

——, *New Tea Lover's Treasury* (San Francisco: Publishing Technology Associates, 1999).

Ody, P., *The Complete Medicinal Herbal* (London: Dorling Kindersley, 1993).

——, *Home Herbal* (London: Dorling Kindersley, 1995).

Oppliger, P., *Green Tea: The Delicious Everyday Health Drink* (Essex, UK: C. W. Daniel Company Limited, 1998).

Quimme, P., *Coffee and Tea* (New York: Signet, 1976).

Republic of Tea, *The Book of Tea and Herbs* (Santa Rosa, CA: Cole Group, 1993).

Rosen, D., *Steeped in Tea* (Pownal, VT: Storey Books, 1999).

Schafer, C., and Shafer, V., *Teacraft* (San Francisco: Yerba Buena Press, 1975).

Sen XV, S., *Tea Life, Tea Mind* (New York: Weatherhill, 1981).

Slavin, S., and Petzke, K., *Tea Essence of the Leaf* (San Francisco: Chronicle Books, 1998).

Smith, M., *The Afternoon Tea Book* (New York: Atheneum, 1986).

Weiner, M. A., and Weiner, J. A., *Herbs That Heal* (Mill Valley, CA: Quantum Books, 1994).

Wild, A., *The East India Company Book of Tea* (London: HarperCollins, 1994).

Zak, V., *20,000 Secrets of Tea* (New York: Dell, 1999).

Articles (from print and online sources)

"The Benefits of Green Tea," by Joseph Contorno, *Les Nouvelles Esthétiques,* July 1997.

"A Bit of Science . . . on the Subject of Tea," Coffeetea.about.com.

"A Cup of Tea," December 17, 1998, Healing.about.com.

"Drinking Tea May Help You Lose Weight," by L. A. McKeown, March 22, 2000, WebMD Medical News.

"For British Ladies, Afternoon Tea Appears to Help Prevent Osteoporosis," by Jeanie Davis, April 13, 2000, WebMD Medical News.

"Good Health in a Cup," Herbsforhealth.com.

"Green Tea May Really Work on Skin," by Deeann Glamser, August 15, 2000, OnehealthMD.com.

"Green Tea Good for Your Skin?" by Renee Libutti, January 22, 2001, WABC.

Notes

"Green Tea Battles Arthritis," by Katrina Woznicky, July 26, 1999, WebMD Medical News.

"Green Tea Could Be Good for Your Skin, Study Finds," by Andrea M. Braslavsky, August 17, 2000, WebMD Medical News.

"Green Tea Extract Fights Cancer," by Holly McCord, Women.com.

"The Healing Powers of Tea," by Mindy Hermann, *Family Circle,* June 1, 1999.

"The Health Benefits of Drinking Green Tea," About.com.

"Healthy Bodycare," by Susan Lacroix, Alternativemedicine.com.

"Heart-Healthy Tea," 2000, WholeHealthMD.com.

"Ingredients in Green Tea Can Protect Against Cancer, Heart Disease," by Mike Fillon, December 2, 1999, WebMD Medical News.

"The Miracle of Green Tea," About.com.

"News on the Health Benefits of Tea, Presented by John H. Weisburger, American Health Foundation, Valhalla, NY," February 1999, Tinyteapot.com.

"Research Suggests Tea Might Be Good for the Heart," November 14, 2000, CNN.com.

"Scientists Uncover New Cancer-Fighting Benefits in Tea," American Institute for Cancer Research, December 7, 1999.

"Scientists Gather to Report Benefits of Tea," by Katrina Woznicki, September 15, 1998, Onhealth.webmd.com.

"South African Antioxidant Tea Can Help Build a Better Immune System," *Hanford Sentinel,* May 30, 2000.

"Strongest of All Antioxidants Found in Green Tea," Tea & Health News Center, April 25, 1999, Greentea.com.

"Tea Research Association Establishes Tea As Health Drink," March 6, 1997, Business Line & Tribeca Internet Initiatives, Inc.

"Tea Time," by Sandy Laurie, Vegsource.com.

"Teasing Out Tea's Hearty-Healthy Effect," *Science News,* vol. 158, December 2, 2000.

"Tea's Anti-Cancer Role Challenged," March 5, 1996, Onhealth.webmd.com.

"Tea's Reputation As a Healthy Brew Increasing," by Sue Licher, June 19, 2000, CNN.com.

"Weak Tea As Strong Medicine," by Carla Helfferich, January 8, 1992, Healing.about.com.

NOTES

Websites

Celestial Seasonings (www.celestialseasonings.com)
Lipton Tea (www.liptont.com)
Tea Council of Canada (www.tea.ca)
The Tea Pages (www.teatime.com)
United Kingdom Tea Council (www.teahealth.co.uk)
Urasenke Konnichian (www.urasenke.or.jp)

Press Kits and Fact Sheets

Bigelow
Five Roses
Good Earth Products
Lipton's Tea & Health Information Center
The Republic of Tea
Rooibos Ltd.
Second International Scientific Symposium on Tea & Human Health
The Stash Tea Company
Taylors of Harrogate
The Tea Council of the USA
Traditional Medicinals

Index

Index

INDEX

THE LITTLE PILATES BOOK

Flatten your stomach, tone your thighs, and get rid of love handles—without doing crunches! A holistic exercise designed to condition body and mind, pilates helps strengthen core muscles, improve posture, reduce lower back pain, and increase flexibility for a strong, supple body. Complete with easy-to-follow instructions and illustrations, *The Little Pilates Book* is the perfect introduction to this dynamic mat-exercise program.

THE LITTLE FOOT CARE BOOK

If you've ever uttered the words "My feet are killing me!" you need this book. This fun, concise guide will teach you how to pamper your feet and enjoy the total body benefits of good foot health—even when you're always on the go. With its easy-to-follow advice, it shows you how to soothe your aching feet to reduce stress, promote relaxation, and restore energy. So take the right step with *The Little Foot Care Book*.